Designing Safe Housing Environments for Older Adults

Older adults spend a large part of their lives in their homes and carry out important tasks within them. According to social determinants of health, the built environment is one of five topics that affect health and quality of life. With population aging coming into focus, designing safe home environments for older adults is a topic of serious discussion. The physical characteristics of the environment have a direct impact on the comfort and confidence of users and can significantly influence the aging process. This book addresses the key issues to consider when focusing on the design for safe and comfortable living for older adults.

Presenting design strategies for housing environments for older adults based on the concepts of aging in place, human factors, and safety, it covers topics such as activities of daily living, independence, autonomy and dependence, risk factors for falls, types of environmental adaptations, and safe housing. Design solutions are offered, and each housing space reveals explanations and ideas for improving activities for residents. Split into two sections, the book takes a theoretical approach that provides notes about important concepts that need to be learned before starting the project or adapting a housing environment. It then shows the practical measures that are necessary to be implemented in environments, based on the level of safety. The reader will obtain a full and thorough knowledge of the key design considerations to deliver retrofits and new ideas to existing properties.

Designing Safe Housing Environments for Older Adults is an ideal read for professionals in the fields of health and safety, ergonomics and human factors, designers, civil engineers, architects, and interior designers.

Juliana Tasca Tissot is Professor of Faculty of Architecture at the Federal University of Pelotas, Brazil. She has a bachelor, master's, and PhD degree in architecture. She was Visiting Scholar at the University of Illinois supervised by Dr. Wendy Rogers in the Department of Kinesiology and Community Health in 2022. She is certified as an Aging in Place Specialist by NAHB. Her research interests include design for aging with a focus on the built environment. She also studies the relationship between the reduction of falls, usability of the space, accessibility, and healthy aging.

Human Factors and Aging Series

Series Editor: Wendy A. Rogers, University of Illinois Urbana-Champaign

Given the worldwide aging of the population, there is a tremendous increase in system, environment, and product designs targeted to the older population. The purpose of this series is to provide focused volumes on different topics of human factors/ergonomics as they affect design for older adults. The books are translational in nature meaning that they are accessible to a broad audience of readers. The target audience includes human factors/ergonomics specialists, gerontologists, psychologists, health-related practitioners, as well as industrial designers. The unifying theme of the books is the relevance and contributions of the field of human factors to design for an aging population.

Designing Telehealth for an Aging Population: A Human Factors Perspective
Neil Charness, George Demiris, Elizabeth Krupinski

Designing Training and Instructional Programs for Older Adults
Sara J. Czaja, Joseph Sharit

Designing Technology Training for Older Adults in Continuing Care Retirement Communities
Shelia R. Cotten, Elizabeth A. Yost, Ronald W. Berkowsky, Vicki Winstead, William A. Anderson

Designing for Older Adults: Principles and Creative Human Factors Approaches, Third Edition
Sara J. Czaja, Walter R. Boot, Neil Charness, Wendy A. Rogers

Designing Transportation Systems for Older Adults
Carryl L. Baldwin, Bridget A. Lewis, Pamela M. Greenwood

Designing Displays for Older Adults, Second Edition
Anne McLaughlin, Richard Pak

Designing for Older Adults: Case Studies, Methods, and Tools
Walter Boot, Neil Charness, Sara J Czaja, Wendy A. Rogers

Designing Robots to Improve Quality of Life for Older Adults
Wendy A. Rogers and Tracy L. Mitzner

Designing Safe Housing Environments for Older Adults
Juliana Tasca Tissot

For more information about this series, please visit: www.crcpress.com/Human-Factors-and-Aging-Series/book-series/CRCHUMFACAGI

Designing Safe Housing Environments for Older Adults

Juliana Tasca Tissot

CRC Press
Taylor & Francis Group
Boca Raton London New York

CRC Press is an imprint of the
Taylor & Francis Group, an **informa** business

First edition published 2026
by CRC Press
2385 NW Executive Center Drive, Suite 320, Boca Raton FL 33431

and by CRC Press
4 Park Square, Milton Park, Abingdon, Oxon, OX14 4RN

CRC Press is an imprint of Taylor & Francis Group, LLC

ISBN: 978-1-032-89618-2 (hbk)
ISBN: 978-1-032-89463-8 (pbk)
ISBN: 978-1-003-54370-1 (ebk)

DOI: 10.1201/9781003543701

Typeset in Times
by Apex CoVantage, LLC

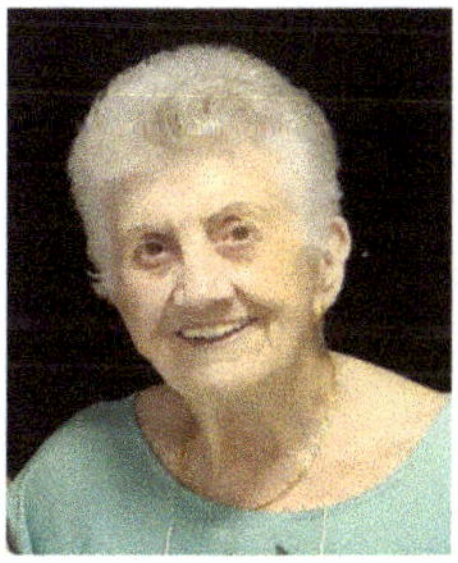

I dedicate this book to my beloved grandmother—Nelcy T. Z. Tasca, whose strength, vitality, and example of independent living inspire me deeply. Her love and life journey form the foundation of my sensitive and committed perspective in seeking strategies that promote more comfortable environments, addressing the needs and aspirations of older adults, and enabling them to age with independence and safety in their own homes.

Contents

Preface

This book was born out of a personal concern: how can we create living environments that are truly safe, welcoming, and capable of promoting the independence of older adults in their daily lives? In the context of a rapidly aging population where older adults remain increasingly active, there is an urgent need to rethink residential spaces so that they keep pace with these new ways of living. As an architect, I have always been deeply touched by this reality, reflecting on how spaces can be designed to enable people to live better lives.

Throughout my academic journey, I conducted research that helped me find ways to answer these questions, including my dissertation. Based on the results I obtained, I felt the need to ensure that this knowledge could reach as many people as possible and that the outcomes could truly help create safer homes for older adults. This book emerged as a tool to guide and contribute to that purpose. The primary goal of this book is to serve as a practical guide for a diverse readership: professionals involved in the design and renovation of spaces, as well as individuals who wish to adapt their own homes or the homes of their family members.

On each page, there is a commitment to providing practical and evidence-based guidance that enables homes to become safer, more comfortable, and capable of sustaining independence, which are so essential to well-being in later life. I hope this work contributes to the development of projects that are more sensitive to the real needs of older adults, inspiring transformations in the ways we design, adapt, and live in spaces over time.

Numerous people in both my professional and personal life have supported my efforts to complete this book. While I list their names here, words cannot fully express the depth of my gratitude for their contributions:

- Wendy A. Rogers, for her insightful guidance and thoughtful reviews of early chapter drafts.
- The members of the Human Factors & Aging Laboratory, for their support and collaboration throughout my dissertation research.
- CRC Press and our Editor James Hobbs, for their consistent assistance throughout the writing process.
- My family and friends, for their continued support, patience, and encouragement every step of the way.
- Lizandra G. Lupi Vergara, for assisting me during my dissertation journey.
- Christy McGuire, for her careful editing and invaluable feedback.

The book is intended for a broad audience, including gerontologists, human factors and ergonomics specialists, architects, designers, and professionals involved in creating and adapting living environments for all, especially older adults.

Thank you for reading.

—Juliana T. Tissot, PhD

Section I

Theoretical Approach

1 Introduction and Overview

This book should be viewed as a guide to help understand how housing spaces for older adults can support aging in place for as long as possible, with safety, autonomy, and independence. It has been developed based on both theoretical and practical research, which informed a set of guidelines for designing housing spaces for older adults. In this first section, the topics discussed have a more theoretical focus, providing foundational knowledge about the essential concepts necessary to design safer environments for this population.

The housing environment is crucial in the lives of older adults, influencing not only their daily routines but also their overall well-being and quality of life. As people age, their relationship with their home becomes more complex, shaped by their changing physical, emotional, and social needs. Understanding the factors that affect the use of housing environments by older adults requires an exploration of several key concepts including place attachment, activities of daily living (ADLs), and the critical notions of independence, autonomy, and dependence; concepts about aging in place; and safe housing and risk factors for falls. These concepts are deeply interconnected and have significant implications for how homes are designed to support aging in place.

The place attachment, the emotional bond that individuals form with their living spaces, is an essential aspect of aging in place. For older adults, the home is often more than just a physical space; it represents comfort, familiarity, history, and a sense of security. The meaning attached to one's home can significantly affect their desire to remain in it as they age. Understanding this attachment is crucial when considering the design of environments that promote aging in place, as it shapes how individuals experience their daily lives and interact with their surroundings.

Equally important are the activities of daily living (ADLs), which encompass the fundamental tasks individuals perform to care for themselves and maintain their independence. The concepts of independence, autonomy, and dependence are central to understanding how housing can impact older adults, and these concepts should play a critical role when designing environments that support older adults in maintaining their dignity and self-sufficiency.

The physical environment can either support or hinder an individual's ability to age independently and with dignity. Aging is accompanied by a range of biological, behavioral, economic, and environmental factors that influence an older adult's ability to live safely and independently in their home. One of the most significant risks older adults face is the danger of falls, which are a leading cause of injury and loss of independence. Fall risk factors include biological factors, such as decreased muscle strength and balance; behavioral factors, such as medication use or lack of physical activity; economic factors, such as limited resources for home modifications; and

DOI: 10.1201/9781003543701-2

environmental factors, such as poor lighting or hazardous flooring. Understanding these risks is vital in designing homes that not only accommodate the needs of older adults but also actively reduce the potential for falls.

The concepts explored in the first section lay the foundation for understanding how to create safer, more supportive housing environments for older adults. Topics such as place attachment, activities of daily living (ADLs), aging in place, and fall risk factors provide essential insights into the needs and challenges faced by this population. These concepts highlight the intricate relationship between individuals and their homes, emphasizing the importance of designing environments that foster safety, independence, and well-being. At the end of this section, seven categories that address the key elements of a home environment will be explored in detail to provide a comprehensive approach to creating homes that support aging in place while enhancing safety, independence, and well-being.

In the following four chapters, these theoretical discussions will transition into practical applications. Section Two of this book will build upon these concepts and present detailed guidelines for designing specific spaces within the home, offering actionable strategies to address the needs identified in this section.

2 Aspects That Influence the Use of Housing Space by Older Adults

2.1 PLACE ATTACHMENT

There are several factors that influence older adults' desire to remain in their homes as they age, with place attachment being a significant one. For older adults, the concept of home is multifaceted, encompassing perspectives related to both security and freedom. From their viewpoint, home is at the core of their identity and is a source of enduring care. The home environment holds deep meanings tied to personal experiences, life history, and personality.

According to Nygren et al. (2007), the concept of home integrates subjective evaluations, values, cognitions, and emotions, reflecting a person's relationship with their living space. The connection between older adults and their homes is a profound expression of their identity, shaped by personal and meaningful elements that contribute to their sense of protection and well-being. Having a space under their own control offers numerous advantages such as freedom, independence, and the ability to live on their own terms. Living on one's own terms includes engaging in activities at their preferred pace, watching their favorite television programs at chosen times, pursuing hobbies, traveling, and interacting with neighbors without fear of judgment or interference from family members (Tomazzoni, 2011).

When designing physical environments centering the concept of aging in place, it is essential to understand the meaning of place attachment, which is closely tied to prolonged exposure to a specific location. This attachment significantly shapes how meaning is attributed to the spaces inhabited and used by older adults. Another aspect related to place attachment is place identity, which emerges through a combination of memories, perceptions, interpretations, ideas, and emotions associated with physical environments. In this sense, a place is not merely a physical space but a socially constructed environment imbued with social and emotional significance (Phillips et al., 2011).

Furthermore, emotions are a vital aspect of human life, profoundly influencing how we make decisions, assess risks, solve problems, direct our attention, identify points of interest, and categorize information. Spaces that generate positive emotions can encourage users to spend more time in them. These positive emotional responses are essential for enhancing the well-being of older adults, contributing significantly to their overall health and quality of life (Lee & Kim, 2020).

In summary, the concepts of place attachment, home, and the emotional resonance of spaces are deeply interconnected and play a critical role in the well-being

DOI: 10.1201/9781003543701-3

of older adults. A home is more than just a physical structure—it is a space imbued with personal meaning shaped by memories, experiences, and emotional connections that foster a sense of identity and autonomy. Positive emotional responses to well-designed spaces can enhance an individual's quality of life, encouraging aging in place and promoting independence. By understanding these dynamics, we can create environments that support the practical needs of older adults and nurture their emotional and psychological well-being, empowering them to thrive as they age.

2.2 ACTIVITIES OF DAILY LIVING

Activities of daily living (ADLs) play a central role in the lives of older adults, serving as essential indicators of their ability to maintain independence and quality of life. These activities encompass a wide range of tasks that support physical well-being, social engagement, and participation within the community. For older individuals, the ability to carry out these activities can often reflect their overall health, functionality, and autonomy. Understanding the specific needs and challenges related to ADLs is crucial for creating environments that support aging in place and promote safety, dignity, and well-being.

In daily routines at home, individuals engage in various ADLs, which are used to assess a person's ability to live independently. Lawton and Brody (1969) developed categories to assess the functional status of older adults, helping to identify levels of independence and care needs. This classification has since become a standard tool for health professionals, researchers, and caregivers in evaluating aging individuals' capacities and designing appropriate interventions. These categories are as follows:

Basic activities of daily living (BADLs) are essential self-care tasks that individuals must perform to maintain physical health and well-being. For older adults, these activities often serve as benchmarks for assessing their ability to live independently and their overall functional capacity.

BADLs are fundamental to daily life and typically include the following:

- Eating and drinking: the ability to feed oneself, including preparing simple meals, using utensils, and managing hydration. For older adults, challenges such as arthritis, swallowing difficulties, or dental problems may require adaptive tools or dietary modifications.
- Bathing and personal hygiene: these tasks include taking a shower or bath, washing hair, brushing teeth, and other grooming activities. For older adults with mobility issues or balance concerns, features like grab bars, non-slip bath mat, and walk-in tubs can be essential for safety.
- Dressing: the ability to select appropriate clothing for the weather or occasion and to physically put on and take off garments. Adaptive clothing can assist those with limited dexterity or mobility.
- Toileting: managing personal hygiene during and after using the restroom, which includes getting to and from the toilet, transferring safely, and cleaning oneself. Modifications such as raised toilet seats and bidet attachments can enhance independence and comfort.

- Mobility: moving safely within one's living space, including getting in and out of bed, sitting down or standing up, and walking short distances. Mobility aids like canes, walkers and rollators, or wheelchairs may be necessary for individuals with limited physical strength or balance issues.

BADLs are critical not only for an individual's independence but also for their sense of self-worth and quality of life. When older adults face challenges in performing these tasks, caregivers and designers must focus on solutions that promote autonomy, such as assistive devices, ergonomic design features, and personalized care plans. Ensuring that older adults can continue to perform their BADLs safely and effectively is a fundamental part of supporting their overall well-being.

Instrumental activities of daily living (IADLs) refers to complex tasks that enable older adults to live independently within their communities. Unlike BADLs, which focus on fundamental self-care, IADLs involve activities that support independence and allow individuals to manage their lives outside of basic personal needs.

These tasks are often indicators of an older adult's ability to function in a broader social and community context. The ability to perform IADLs is a critical aspect of assessing an individual's overall health and autonomy.

Some types of IADLs include the following:

- Meal preparation: the ability to plan and prepare meals includes selecting healthy foods, cooking, and managing dietary needs. Older adults with mobility issues, cognitive decline, or vision impairment may need adaptive kitchen tools or assistance with meal planning.
- Managing finances: handling personal finances such as paying bills, budgeting, and managing bank accounts are vital for independence.
- Shopping: includes the ability to go grocery shopping, purchase household items, and manage a shopping list. Older adults may require assistance with transportation, carrying heavy items, or using online shopping platforms as an alternative.
- Housekeeping: maintaining a clean and safe living environment, including tasks such as laundry, cleaning, and organizing.
- Transportation: the ability to use public transportation, drive a car, or arrange for rides to appointments and social events is crucial for community participation.
- Medication management: taking the right medications at the right time is critical for health. IADLs in this category involve managing prescriptions, understanding dosages, and remembering to take medications. Pill organizers, medication reminders, or caregiver support can help older adults stay on track with their health regimens.
- Communication: the ability to use a telephone, computer, or other means to communicate with others is essential for social engagement and accessing services. For some older adults, adapting to new technology or using assistive devices like hearing aids or speech-to-text software can help maintain communication with loved ones and healthcare providers.

IADLs are not only crucial for an older adult's independence but also for maintaining a connection to the outside world and their community. Difficulty in performing these tasks can indicate a need for increased support, whether through technology, caregivers, or modifications to the living environment. By addressing these needs, it is possible to enhance the autonomy, safety, and quality of life for older adults.

Another category that is important to mention about ADLs is **enhanced activities of daily living (EADLs),** which refers to activities that go beyond basic self-care and functional tasks, aiming to support older adults in maintaining an active, fulfilling lifestyle. This category was highlighted in research conducted by Rogers et al. (1998).

Enhanced activities of daily living (EADLs) can be defined as social and recreational activities that contribute to an older adult's emotional and psychological well-being. These activities go beyond basic needs and help foster a sense of purpose, connection, and enjoyment in life.

EADLs are essential for maintaining an active and fulfilling lifestyle, supporting mental health, and preventing feelings of isolation. Socialization and leisure activities allow older adults to engage with their communities, nurture relationships, and continue to develop personal interests.

Some examples of EADLs include the following:

- Socializing with friends and family: regular interactions with friends, family, and neighbors are crucial for combating loneliness and maintaining social bonds. Activities like having guests over for a meal, attending family gatherings, or meeting friends for coffee help older adults stay socially connected and engaged.
- Participating in group activities or clubs: joining clubs, senior centers, or hobby groups allows older adults to share common interests with others. For example, attending a book club, participating in a knitting group, or joining a walking or gardening club can provide both social interaction and mental stimulation.
- Attending religious or spiritual services: for many older adults, attending religious or spiritual services is an important part of their routine, offering a sense of community and spiritual fulfillment. Participating in prayer groups, church activities, or community volunteer projects can be integral to their social engagement.
- Pursuing hobbies and personal interests: engaging in hobbies such as painting, music, photography, or gardening provides older adults with a sense of accomplishment and enjoyment. Whether learning a new craft, attending a painting class, or gardening in the backyard, these activities offer mental stimulation and emotional satisfaction.
- Exercising and physical activities: physical engagement is a key component of EADLs, with activities like walking, swimming, dancing, or yoga helping older adults stay active, improve their health, and interact with others. Many senior centers and community organizations offer fitness classes designed for older adults, fostering both physical and social well-being.
- Receiving friends and visitors at home: the ability to host and engage with others in a social setting such as receiving people at home is a vital social

activity that contributes to emotional well-being and helps maintain strong social bonds. For older adults, the opportunity to invite family, friends, or neighbors into their home provides social interaction, sense of purpose, and connection to the outside world.

EADLs are essential for promoting mental and emotional health in older adults. Social interaction, engaging in meaningful activities, and having opportunities for recreation and fun all contribute to a richer, more fulfilling life. By encouraging older adults to participate in EADLs, we help them maintain a sense of identity, self-worth, and connection to the world around them, which are crucial for their overall well-being.

When designing a safe and functional home environment, it is crucial to evaluate the activities that individuals perform and identify any challenges they may encounter. Living alone can pose additional risks for older adults, as it increases their vulnerability to accidents, given that they must complete all tasks independently. However, it is important to recognize that the built environment can play a significant role in mitigating and even preventing these risks through thoughtful design strategies. It is essential to consider the interplay between an individual's abilities, the activities they engage in, and the environment itself. By addressing these factors together, we can create spaces that promote safety, minimize accidents, and support overall well-being.

When considering the housing needs of older adults, it is vital to integrate the design of living spaces with their daily activities. A supportive environment that considers the physical, cognitive, and emotional aspects of ADLs enables older adults to age in place safely, independently, and with a higher quality of life. The more the home environment can accommodate these activities—whether through accessibility features, safety modifications, or spaces for social interaction—the more it supports the well-being of older adults. Ultimately, creating a home that is both functional and conducive to aging in place is essential for promoting health, autonomy, and happiness in the later stages of life.

2.3 INDEPENDENCE, AUTONOMY, AND DEPENDENCY

The design of a safe and functional living environment is grounded in several key principles and concepts. One of the key points to consider in planning safe environments for older adults is assessing the user's level of independence, autonomy, or dependence. This evaluation is crucial for understanding the individual's abilities, limitations, and specific needs, which in turn guides the development of an environment that supports their well-being.

Independence, autonomy, and dependence are distinct yet interconnected concepts that reflect how a person interacts with their environment and carries out daily tasks. Recognizing these different levels helps designers create spaces that accommodate everyone's unique requirements. For example, an independent person may require minimal modifications to their home, while someone with more limited autonomy may benefit from features that promote greater ease of movement and decision-making. Understanding these nuances is essential for developing environments that ensure safety, sense of dignity, and empowerment for the user.

Independence is the ability to perform daily life activities without the need for assistance from others. It involves managing one's personal care, chores, and tasks autonomously. Some examples are as follows:

- A person feels thirsty, so they get up, walk to the kitchen, open the fridge, and pour themselves a glass of water.
- They can cook a simple meal, such as making a sandwich or preparing a salad, without needing help.
- They can clean and maintain their living space such as sweep the floor or make the bed on their own.
- They independently manage personal hygiene tasks like brushing their teeth or taking a shower.

In essence, independence means having the physical and cognitive ability to manage one's environment and routine without relying on others. This autonomy contributes to a sense of self-sufficiency and control over daily life.

Autonomy is the ability to make personal decisions about how to live daily life, based on one's own preferences, values, and needs. It involves having control over one's actions and choices, even if physical or cognitive limitations may affect the ability to carry out those decisions independently. Some examples are as follows:

- A person may recognize that they are thirsty and want to drink water, but due to physical limitations, they may require assistance to reach or pour the water.
- An individual may decide what to wear each day based on their personal style and comfort, but may need help dressing due to mobility issues.
- A person may choose their daily activities such as deciding to read, exercise, or socialize, but they may need modifications in the environment or assistance to engage in these activities.
- Someone may plan their day, decide on meals, or manage their finances based on personal preferences, but may rely on adaptive tools or support to carry out those tasks.

Autonomy is about maintaining the freedom to make decisions that reflect one's own desires and needs, even if some aspects of daily life require external support. It reflects a person's ability to govern their life according to their own rules and preferences, even when faced with challenges.

Dependence refers to the inability to perform daily life activities without assistance from others. It occurs when an individual's physical, cognitive, or emotional limitations prevent them from carrying out essential tasks independently. Dependence can vary in degree, ranging from needing occasional support to requiring full assistance with most activities. Some examples are as follows:

- A person may be unable to walk or move around their home without the aid of a caregiver or mobility device, such as a wheelchair or walker.
- They may need help with personal hygiene tasks such as bathing, dressing, or grooming, due to limited mobility or dexterity.

- A person may be unable to prepare meals or manage household chores independently and require assistance with cooking, cleaning, or shopping.
- They may rely on someone to help manage their medications, ensuring they take the correct dosage at the right time.
- An individual might need help with basic decision-making or managing finances such as paying bills due to cognitive impairments like dementia.

Dependence highlights the need for support systems to ensure the individual's well-being and safety, emphasizing the importance of tailored environments and care services to meet their specific needs.

Many people maintain their autonomy (decision-making capacity) even though they are dependent (physically incapable of performing a certain action). Some illnesses or accidents can mean that people can choose, for example, what clothes they want to wear, but they are not actually able to perform such a task.

The design of a housing environment can significantly contribute to enhancing the independence, autonomy, and well-being of older adults while helping to reduce dependence on external help. A well-designed home can create a space that allows older adults to perform daily tasks independently and/or with minimal assistance, offering opportunities for personal decision-making and control over their lives.

To promote independence, the housing space should be free from barriers that hinder mobility, such as narrow doorways or uneven flooring. Features like wide hallways, non-slip floors, and accessible furniture allow for greater ease of movement and help prevent accidents.

Autonomy can be fostered through a home environment that encourages choice and self-expression. Spaces that can be personalized—whether through adjustable furniture, multifunctional areas, or spaces designed for relaxation and leisure—allow older adults to maintain a sense of control over how they live.

At the same time, the built environment can reduce dependence by ensuring that the person can remain safe and secure within their home. The addition of safety features such as grab bars, proper lighting, and fall-prevention measures helps mitigate the risk of accidents and increases the confidence with which older adults can move about their homes.

When designed with the needs of older adults in mind, the housing environment plays a crucial role in enhancing their independence and autonomy. It allows them to maintain control over their lives and daily routines, reduces the risk of accidents, and helps to minimize reliance on external assistance. Integrating thoughtful design solutions, can create environments that empower older adults to live safely, confidently, and with dignity in their own homes.

This chapter highlights key concepts for promoting the well-being of older adults in their living environments. By addressing these aspects, housing environments can be designed to empower older adults to live with dignity, confidence, and control over their daily lives. For developing clear guidelines for housing design, it is important to learn about these principles. Such guidelines can ensure that living environments address the practical needs of older adults while promoting their emotional and psychological well-being.

3 Concepts About Housing and Aging

3.1 AGING AND ARCHITECTURE

Aging is a multifaceted process that encompasses molecular, cellular, behavioral, cognitive, and social factors, which are intrinsic to the human cycle of life (Cruz & Leite, 2018). With the increase in the global population of older adults, the importance of addressing aging has grown considerably across various fields including architecture. The intersection between aging and architecture represents a promising field in professional activity and research area due to the need to create adequate, functional, and safe environments for older adults. Changes in physical and cognitive abilities in addition to the barriers in the environment can be a challenge for those who wish to remain in their home while they age (age in place).

In this sense, architecture for aging emerges, which considers design environments that meet present and future needs for increasing the probability of greater independence, autonomy, and quality of life for older adults at home. The physical characteristics of the built environment have a direct impact on the safety, comfort, and confidence of users. The design of living environments must consider design strategies aligned with the concepts of architecture for aging to provide environments compatible with users' needs to improve aging in place.

Quality of life is related to the level of satisfaction and well-being that certain spaces provide. However, due to the physical and cognitive changes these users may experience, certain environmental characteristics can become barriers to performing activities of daily living, directly affecting the usability of the space. Therefore, for a home to be considered adequate, designers must ensure that the environment can compensate for potential health declines that affect individuals as they age, allowing tasks to be carried out with comfort and safety (Miguel et al., 2018).

In conclusion, aging is a complex process that affects various aspects of life, requiring thoughtful consideration in many fields, especially architecture. The need to create environments that support the physical, cognitive, and social needs of older adults is becoming increasingly important as the global population ages. Architecture for aging aims to address these challenges by designing spaces that promote independence, safety, and well-being for older adults.

The physical environment plays a crucial role in enabling older adults to maintain autonomy and quality of life. Housing spaces must be adapted to accommodate these shifts, minimizing risks such as falls while simultaneously enhancing comfort. Accessibility, flexibility, and user-centered design are vital strategies to ensure that environments evolve with the changing needs of their users.

DOI: 10.1201/9781003543701-4

3.2 AGING IN PLACE

3.2.1 Concept of Aging in Place

Aging in place is defined as the ability to age in a stable environment in which people can maintain independent living circumstances in their own homes (Phillips et al., 2011; Porto & Rezende, 2016). Strategies to provide opportunities for aging in place benefit the entire population as they promote the strengthening of intergenerational relationships between older adults and the community in which they live (Farber & Shinkle, 2011). However, due to the physical and cognitive changes that occur with advancing age, it is essential to have a better understanding of how space interacts with older adults (Hazin, 2012).

The environment in which older adults live should be designed considering personal expectations, cultural aspects, aesthetics, standards, functionality, safety, and the economic conditions of those who live there. Designing an environment suitable for them implies, at the same time, observing all these aspects without impeding the social use of other individuals in any way. Only by this process will we work towards enabling the interaction of the person, with all their characteristics, and the environment in which they live (Romeiro et al., 2010).

As health declines, environmental limitations increasingly conflict with individual abilities, leading to challenges in the interaction between the user and their surroundings and negatively impacting well-being. These challenges underscore the need for environmental adaptations to reduce risks, particularly the risk of falls among older adults (Bhidayasiri et al., 2015). In this context, the home can be understood as a space that mediates the relationship between functional capacity, personal factors, and the physical environment—a concept known as the person-environment approach. This framework encompasses key issues such as housing accessibility and dependence on daily living activities within the home.

The occurrence of falls is directly associated with age and difficulty walking, as the aging process has repercussions on structural and functional changes that modify the pattern of mobility and the individual's relationship with the environment. As the years progress, the importance of environmental factors grows in understanding how older adults perform their social relationships and daily interactions as well as the different ways of becoming ill and the negative health outcomes. In the absence of an environment that optimizes their potential, older adults end up limiting their ability to perform activities, which, within a series of events, ends up fueling changes arising from the biological aging process (Cruz & Leite, 2018).

The appropriate combination between the user and the physical environment generates a more adequate performance in relation to the activities of daily living for older adults, hence the importance of understanding the behavior of people and their spaces, especially in old age. The interaction between the person and the space describes how older adults adapt to the environments to achieve this combination between competence and environment (Leiva-Caro et al., 2015).

Despite many challenges imposed by the conditions of the built environment, interventions in the physical space are less common than adjustments between the user and their behavior in relation to the environment, which would not be ideal.

There are opportunities for interventions in the built environment to help older adults successfully carry out their activities of daily living and thus age in their homes with greater safety and autonomy (Ramadhani & Rogers, 2022).

Solutions based on architecture and design increase the possibility for older adults having a safer living environment in the same space to which they are used to and, therefore, allow them to live longer. To this end, technological interventions are important, as well as interventions related to the physical space (Lee & Kim, 2020; Lien et al., 2015).

The design of home spaces has a significant effect on air distribution, acoustic quality, natural ventilation, and the amount of daylight—aspects that directly influence the lives of human beings. In addition, spaces can change the patterns of life and behavior of a user. Various experiences felt in spaces depend on the aesthetic, functional, and emotional properties of the spaces (Lien et al., 2015). Cooperation in various fields such as architecture, design, medicine, physiotherapy, physical education, psychology, and others is essential for the development of an intelligent environment to improve the quality of human life.

From a design perspective, there are three groups of older adults:

(i) ambitious, who travel and see the world, have access to the internet.
(ii) domestic, independent inside and outside the home, with access to the internet but dependent for outdoor activities.
(iii) dependent, who need professional and informal care at home, often without access to the internet.

Groups (ii) and (iii) will benefit immediately from design to support their autonomy (Van der Cammen et al., 2017). Group (i) does not yet need support but might like to plan for their future needs.

If housing plays a fundamental role in aging in place, the physical environment is recognized as a leading agent in this phenomenon. Thus, architecture, ergonomics, design, accessibility, and universal design are concepts that can be considered for successful aging. Adapting housing into the direction of older adults' needs while respecting the changes inherent in physical and cognitive abilities becomes necessary so that activities of daily living can be performed comfortably and safely.

3.2.2 Importance of Aging in Place

For older adults, housing and the environment are particularly important due to factors such as accessibility and safety, the financial burden of maintaining a home, and emotional and psychological security that a home provides. Satisfactory environments provide health benefits. In this sense, it is important that, whenever possible, older adults have the possibility of choosing the place where they want to live (Romeiro et al., 2010).

Aging in place is a model that involves adapting the physical environment to the needs and capabilities of older adults to ensure safety, comfort, and well-being. For a population that experiences significant physical and cognitive changes as the years go by, living in an environment that meets these demands is essential for their physical, emotional, and financial health.

There are some aspects related with the importance of aging in place:

- Economy: Aging at home offers economic benefits, both for the residents and for the health system. Remaining in a familiar environment can be more financially viable than opting for long-term care facilities, whose costs can be significantly higher. In addition, aging at home helps to reduce the burden on health services, because people who live in adapted and safe environments tend to suffer fewer accidents and require less intensive medical care.
- Well-being: The relationship between older adults and their home goes beyond practical needs. The home offers a stable emotional base, functioning as a refuge that provides psychological security. Staying in the environment where one has built one's life, shared memories, and created bonds has a positive effect on the mental well-being of the elderly. The ability to choose where to grow old reinforces the feeling of autonomy, something crucial for emotional health. A satisfactory home environment brings health benefits, as it promotes emotional comfort and a sense of belonging, factors that have a direct impact on longevity and quality of life (Romeiro et al., 2010).
- Safety: As age advances, physical and cognitive limitations make environments more challenging. The appropriate combination between the user and the environment is essential to allow better performance in activities of daily living, such as getting up, walking, cooking, or bathing. This adjustment between the individual's demands and the characteristics of the environment promotes not only safety but also autonomy, helping older adults to maintain their freedom and control over their routines.
- Comfort: The home environment offers flexibility for adaptations according to personal needs and preferences, ensuring older adults can control decisions related to their daily comfort and life.
- User-centered design: The concept of aging in place is, above all, user-centered on the individual capabilities and limitations of each elderly person. Each person has unique needs that vary according to their health conditions, mobility, cognition, and personal preferences. Therefore, the environment must be adapted in a personalized way, adjusting the characteristics of the space to ensure better interaction between the individual and the place where they live.

The key to the success of aging in place lies in the balance between the demands of the user and the characteristics of the environment. As older adults face physical or cognitive limitations, the environment needs to be adjusted to compensate for these changes, offering adequate support for daily activities. By creating accessible, safe spaces adapted to individual needs, it is possible to ensure that older adults age with dignity and freedom, maintaining their physical, emotional, and financial health in balance.

3.2.3 Scales of Aging in Place

The concept of aging in place can be applied on three different scales, which vary according to the needs of older adults and the complexity of the adaptations required in the environment. These scales reflect the different stages of aging and the variations in health conditions, autonomy and functionality, which require personalized responses from the environment to ensure the quality of life, safety, and well-being.

These three are described in Figure 3.1.

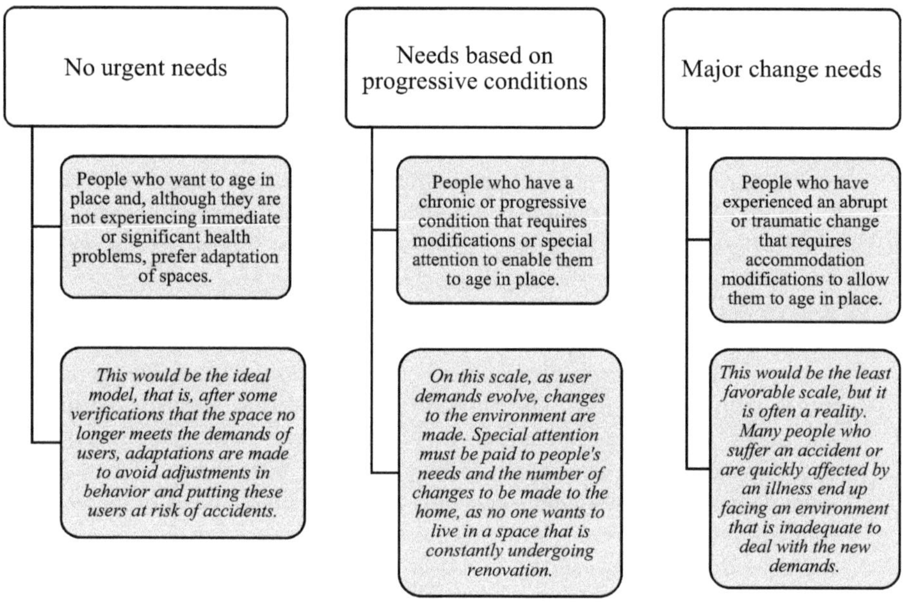

FIGURE 3.1 Scales of aging in place based on human needs.

It is important to know the scales of aging in place because it can help to think and plan the adaptation of spaces throughout our life cycle. Being aware that the environment must be adapted to our needs and not the other way around is already the first step towards more successfully aging in place.

3.3 SAFE HOUSING

There are plenty of characteristics that, when considered into the built environment, can improve the use of the spaces, influencing behavior, habits, and feelings. In addition, it may have a direct impact on the health of residents. Older adults who live in adequate spaces are more satisfied with their environment and, consequently, have better psychological well-being. There are resources aimed at the environment that support the needs of this population and promote their quality of life.

Physical and cognitive abilities can decrease during the aging process; the lower an older adult's ability is, the greater their dependence on the environment will be.

Therefore, the space must be designed with features that facilitate the routine and tasks of users and compensate for such changes.

The design of safe environments must simultaneously promote independence and the feeling of comfort and security. In addition, attention must be paid to anthropometric issues (e.g., reachability and accessibility; mobility and space requirements; strength and dexterity; posture and comfort), which are much more limited in this population. Problems related to the usability of physical space must be solved in relation to both static measurements and those related to the body in movement.

Some reflections and requirements to consider when planning a safe housing:

- Thermal comfort: It is important to highlight that with age, human metabolism suffers a reduction, and as a result, there is a decrease in the amount of water in the organs of the body's skin, which makes older adults colder as well as leads to greater difficulty on adapting to temperature variations (Aihara, 2017). In addition, for physical reasons such as a drop in metabolism, loss of appetite, and poor nutrition, older adults are unable to generate enough heat for the body and therefore are more likely to feel cold. Therefore, with a low level of metabolism and activity, they need a warmer environment with temperature for performing activities is between 68ºF and 73ºF (Hazin, 2012).
- Gradual hearing loss: This type of impairment can cause acoustic comfort levels to change, especially regarding high frequencies, corresponding to high-pitched sounds (Aihara, 2017). With the tendency for hearing capacity to decrease, there is an increase in the production of sounds from radios and television. Thus, the use of thicker walls or internal insulation with appropriate panels helps to minimize the problem (Bestetti, 2006).
- Anthropometric issues: Problems related to the usability of physical space must be solved in relation to both static measurements and those related to the body in movement and must be considered in the design of environments (Daré, 2010). Some examples are maximum and minimum vertical reach (e.g., shelves, cabinets, light switches), horizontal reach limitations (e.g., distance to countertops, appliances), seated vs. standing reach differences (important for wheelchair users); mobility and space with requirements like turning radius for wheelchairs and walkers, clearance width for doorways, hallways, and passageways; strength and dexterity related to grip strength for handles, knobs, and fixtures, finger dexterity for small controls (e.g., buttons, touchscreens), required force to open doors, drawers, or operate devices. Posture and comfort can be seated ergonomics (e.g., seat height, depth, backrest angle), work surface heights for standing and seated users and armrest and footrest positioning.

Another important concept to consider and incorporate into housing projects and adaptations is the concept of universal design. Universal design means the design of products, environments, programs, and services to be used by all people without the need for adaptation or specific design (Mace, 1998). There are seven principles to be considered, as described in Table 3.1.

TABLE 3.1
Principles of Universal Design and Examples of Applications for Aging in Place

Principles	Examples
Equitable use: spaces, objects and products that can be used by people with different abilities, making all environments equal	Entry doors with level access or gentle ramps allow individuals with reduced mobility, such as wheelchair or walker users, to enter the home easily and safely
Flexible use: product design that serves people with different abilities and preferences, being adaptable to any use	Adjustable showers can be easily repositioned or modified to meet the needs of individuals with varying mobility levels
Simple and intuitive use: easy to understand so that anyone can understand it regardless of their experience, knowledge, language ability, or level of concentration	Door handles with lever designs. Unlike traditional round knobs, lever handles are easier to operate, requiring less grip strength and dexterity. They can be easily pushed down with the forearm, elbow, or hand, making them accessible for older adults with arthritis, limited hand strength, or other mobility issues. This simple, intuitive design ensures that doors are easy to open without complicated mechanisms
Easy to perceive information: when the necessary information is transmitted in a way that meets the needs of the recipient, regardless of their knowledge of language or someone with vision or hearing difficulties	Color contrast for areas like light switches, doors, stairs, or hazardous zones. For instance, high-contrast labels or illuminated signs can highlight important areas such as emergency buttons, light switches, or danger warnings
Error tolerance: designed to minimize the risks and possible consequences of accidental or unintentional actions	Presence sensors that automatically turn on or off. Gas sensors detect leaks and shut off gas supply automatically, and smoke detectors help to create a safer living environment
Low physical effort: to be used efficiently, with comfort and minimal fatigue	Built-in shelf, bench, or table located outside the door at the house entrance. This element provides a place to put packages while opening doors, reducing the user's effort when entering the home
Space for approach and use: establishes appropriate dimensions and spaces for access, reach, manipulation, and use, regardless of body size (obese, little person, etc.), posture, or mobility of the user (people in wheelchairs, with strollers, canes etc.)	Appliances and equipment should be within reach of the users, easy to access without requiring them to adapt their behavior in a way that puts them at risk

Source: Based on Mace (1998).

The elements of the built environment can improve or harm human health, influencing behavior, habits, and feelings, and having a direct impact on physical health. Therefore, making health an explicit component of the planning of physical spaces is essential (Lekić et al., 2018). Older adults who live in humanized spaces show greater satisfaction with the environment and psychological well-being (Manca et al., 2019). In addition, researchers have observed significant correlations between specific perceived environmental qualities and general psychological results that confirm the importance of environmental resources to support the needs of older adults and promote their quality of life.

To meet the demands of this age group, some criteria must be included in projects, such as taking care of the low level of personal space, excessive noise, presence of unpleasant odors, inadequate temperature and ventilation, lack of views of green spaces, and insufficient or excessive intensity of artificial lighting.

People are aging, and all aspects of the physical environment including layout and other interfaces must be redesigned to accommodate the needs of this target audience. There is much greater coherence in designing for everyone rather than creating a different or specific design for individuals who have some type of disability, and this is how universal design is conceived.

The concepts presented in this chapter are fundamental for understanding how to design living environments that promote safety, comfort, and well-being for older adults. As the global population ages, the necessity for housing solutions that address the unique physical, cognitive, and emotional needs of older individuals becomes increasingly critical. By incorporating these principles, architects, designers, and planners can create spaces that support independence, reduce risks such as falls, and improve overall satisfaction and health outcomes for older residents.

Moreover, older adults themselves can learn how to enhance their living environments and make adaptations to better support their daily living activities. The application of these strategies ensures that living environments become more functional, accessible, nurturing, and inclusive, allowing older adults to age with dignity and autonomy. This comprehensive approach to housing design not only addresses the immediate needs of older individuals but contributes to a more age-friendly society, where their requirements are met through thoughtful, innovative, and empathetic solutions.

4 Fall Risk Factors

4.1 OVERVIEW OF FALL RISK FACTORS

Fall risk factors are conditions or circumstances that increase the likelihood of a person, especially an older adult, experiencing a fall. The predisposition of factors associated with falls in this population are complex and depend on the characteristics of the individual, their immediate environment, and the interaction between these two.

As people age, their physical abilities may decline, and when combined with factors such as medication use, balance and gait issues, alcohol consumption, inappropriate footwear, and environmental hazards, the risk of an older adult suffering a fall significantly increases.

The consequences of a fall in functional capacity for older adults can be a predictive factor for their quality of life, because this event mainly interferes in the development of the activities of daily living (Fhon et al., 2012), in mental health, and social impacts.

The World Health Organization classifies falls risk factors into four dimensions, as shown in Figure 4.1.

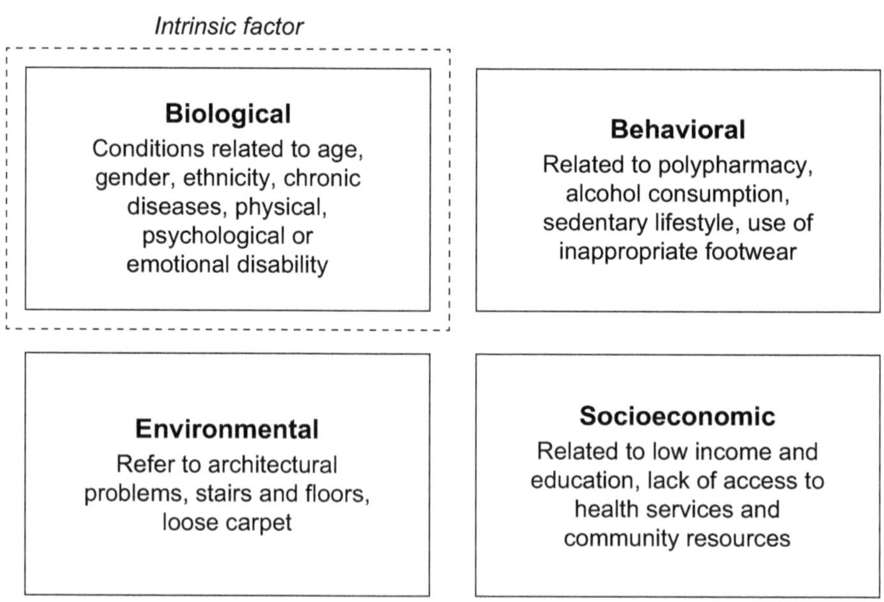

FIGURE 4.1 Fall risk factors based on the World Health Organization.

DOI: 10.1201/9781003543701-5

4.2 BIOLOGICAL

Biological risk factors are those intrinsic to people and reflect disability. They refer to physiological changes related to aging, the presence of acute diseases, muscle weakness, mobility and reaching problems, among others. Physiologically, older adults have a decreased ability to see images with little brightness and color, impairing contrast and visual sharpness. This deficiency has an impact on postural control, as visual information helps to interpret the environment more effectively, allowing safe movements. Visual impairments are an important risk factor for the occurrence of falls, and when associated with other factors, their effect is enhanced (Morais et al., 2012).

The main biological risk factors are as follows:

- Gender.
- Genetic diseases.
- Visual impairments.
- Hearing impairments.
- Cognitive problems.
- Muscle strength.
- Mobility problem.
- Difficulty of reaching high objects, especially for individuals with arthritis or osteoarthritis, as these conditions can limit joint mobility and cause pain, making it challenging to lift arms or stretch.

4.3 BEHAVIORAL

The behavioral risk factor refers to habits, choices, and behaviors that can increase the risk of falls. These behaviors are often related to lifestyle, the way a person performs their activities of daily living and the decisions they make, often without considering the risks associated with age and physical conditions.

The main behavioral risk factors are as follows:

- Neglect in the use of assistive devices.
- Inadequate use of footwear.
- Reckless or excessive physical activities.
- Inappropriate medication.
- Neglecting to adapt to the environment.
- Inattention during activities of daily living.
- Sedentary lifestyle.
- Consumption of alcohol.

4.4 ECONOMICAL

Economic risk factors include aspects related to financial situation and accessibility of resources, which can impact the safety and quality of life of older adults, influencing their housing conditions and care options. It refers to how the financial situation can affect the ability to live safely and independently. When older adults face financial hardship, they may be forced to make decisions that compromise their safety, health, and well-being. This lack of resources can result in inadequate living environments, the inability to purchase necessary products or services, and a reduced quality of life.

The main economic risk factors are as follows:

- Inability to make adaptations to the environment because the financial limited resources.
- Inadequate housing choices.
- Inability to access health and care services.
- Difficulties in purchasing safety equipment.
- Poor diet and lack of nutrients.
- Lack of transportation to social and physical.
- Lack of social interaction and physical inactivity.
- Limited access to community resources.

4.5 ENVIRONMENTAL

Environmental risk factors seem to be the ones most remembered by older adults as causes of falls (Morsch, 2017). Understanding environmental risk factors which are within the individual's control can provide greater safety and a lower risk of falling. Such accidents are observed more frequently among older adults who live alone than among those who live with their family. The risk of domestic accidents among this population is an important public health issue and has a negative effect on the entire family.

Figure 4.2 shows that the rate of YLDs (year lived with disabilities) increases significantly with age, with notable peaks in the older age groups, especially from the age of 60 onwards. Injuries such as hip and femur fractures, as well as severe injuries, are more prevalent in older age groups, indicating an increased vulnerability to severe injuries among this population. Even when a fall does not result in death, it can lead to serious complications affecting morbidity and quality of life.

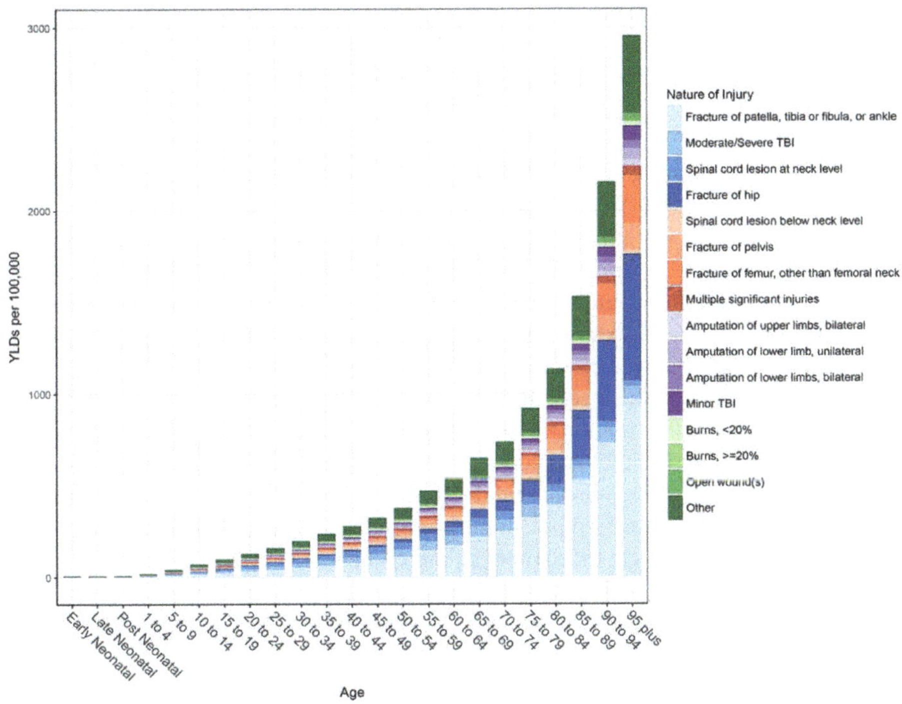

FIGURE 4.2 Age-specific nature-of-injury composition of falls globally.

Source: Spencer L James et al. Inj Prev 2020;26: i3-i11.

Identifying environmental risk factors enables intervention to eliminate these factors and prevent falls. Excessive objects and furniture, associated with insufficient lighting in the environment, increase the number of falls by making it difficult for the individual to interpret the space. Preventing falls is directly related to the reduction or elimination of these factors.

The main environmental risk factors are as follows:

- Carpets.
- Loose threads.
- Steps or uneven surfaces.

- Lack of color contrast.
- Inadequate furniture.
- Inadequate room dimensions for performing activities of daily living.
- Lack of organization and maintenance.
- Dirty.
- Inadequate lighting.

Eliminating or reducing fall risk factors reduces the likelihood of falling. This is very important for older adults who generally have multiple fall risk factors. Risky activities, behaviors, and unsafe environments increase the probability of falling because people can tend to slip, trip, misstep, step incorrectly, and bump into each other, thus creating balance challenges.

The risks depend on the frequency of exposure to the unsafe environment and the functional status of older adults. Environmental risk factors alone may not be enough to cause a fall, but rather the interaction between the abilities of older adults and the degree of exposure to the environmental risk factor are predictive of falls. Therefore, identifying the risk factor is more important than the cause of a fall, because the cause of a fall is a past event that cannot be intervened on, and the risk factors are still present. Preventing falls is directly connected to reducing or eliminating risk factors. As a result, older individuals experience improvements in self-care, which directly impacts their lifestyle and quality of life.

Considering that many physical attributes of the living environment for older adults are linked to fall risks, it is crucial to mitigate these elements. Therefore, in the second section of the book, which focuses on practical approaches, specific characteristics for each area of the home will be presented, based on the safety levels. Since fall risks are associated with a combination of various factors, and the home is where older adults spend a significant portion of their time, reducing these risks can help to prevent potential accidents and enhance the overall quality of life for these individuals.

4.6 RECOMMENDED LINKS

CDC Older adults fall data https://www.cdc.gov/falls/data-research/index.html

SCOR The art & science of risk https://www.scor.com/en/expert-views/falls-are-increasing-among-older-adults

5 Categories for Home Improvement

5.1 OVERVIEW OF CATEGORIES OF HOME IMPROVEMENT

Home improvement refers to modifications and adaptations made to the housing environment with the aim of making it safer, more comfortable, functional, and suitable to the needs of the residents. For older adults, improvements are especially important as they point to increase accessibility, prevent accidents, and facilitate daily living activities.

The adaptations to the built environment have some categories that were developed for this book and vary from cost to time and scope of implementation. They are structural changes, regulations, equipment, assistive technology, construction materials, furniture, and maintenance. Below are the detailed descriptions of each one.

5.2 STRUCTURAL CHANGES

Structural changes refer to deep and permanent modifications made to the housing environment, with the aim of adapting the space to the functional and safety needs of residents. These adjustments require investment of money and time, as they involve more complex aspects of the building as the examples in Table 5.1. Furthermore, for this type of adaptation it is usually necessary to hire a professional from construction to develop the project and supervise the work.

This category of adaptation involves changes to the original structure of the house or apartment, going beyond superficial adaptations, such as installing grab bars or changing furniture. The objective is to transform the environment to ensure accessibility, comfort, and prevent accidents.

TABLE 5.1
Description and Examples of Structural Changes Category

Topic	Description	Example
Removal of architectural barriers	Many houses may have elements that become obstacles to the mobility, such as unevenness between rooms, steps, and narrow passages	Remove internal steps, replacing stairs with ramps or elevators and widening doors and hallways, allowing the passage of wheelchairs and facilitating the use of walkers
Reconfiguration of internal spaces	As people age, the needs for using spaces can change. These structural adjustments ensure that older adults have access to everything they need without having to climb stairs or walk long distances inside the home	Move the bedroom to the ground floor in two-story homes, create an accessible bathroom near the bedroom, and increase the circulation space

(Continued)

DOI: 10.1201/9781003543701-6

TABLE 5.1 *(Continued)*
Description and Examples of Structural Changes Category

Topic	Description	Example
Bathroom adaptations	Bathrooms are high-risk areas for falls and may therefore require significant changes	Installing grab bars, structural changes may include level-free walk-in showers, increasing the circulation space, and installing non-slip flooring
Suitable flooring	The type of flooring used in a home is crucial to the older adults' safety	Replace slippery or uneven flooring with non-slip, easy-to-maintain options, such as vinyl or rubber; level out unevenness between rooms to prevent tripping
Improvements for lighting	Inadequate lighting is harmful to the development of daily living activities and can become a predictor to fall	Increasing the number and size of windows to improve natural lighting, installing additional light points in circulation areas, such as hallways and stairwells

The benefits of structural changes go far outside simple adaptations, offering a range of satisfaction for older adults, their families, and caregivers. It includes prevention of accidents, especially falls, greater independence to perform daily living activities, reduced physical effort for activities, comfort and emotional security, allowing users to live with more confidence.

Structural changes are, therefore, an essential way of adapting the housing environment for healthier and safer aging, ensuring that the home continues to be a place of autonomy and dignity for older adults. It is important to note that in the case of new constructions, the topics outlined in Table 5.1 can be integrated directly into the design. This approach can help avoid costly renovations, as these features are already being accounted for during the planning and construction phases.

5.3 REGULATIONS

Regulations are a set of rules, guidelines, and standards established by competent bodies in each country to ensure the safety, accessibility, and functionality for public and private environments, as will be shown in Table 5.2. These regulations aim to standardize adaptations that make spaces safer and more accessible for users.

Each country and perhaps communities within countries may have a specific set of standards and laws that determine how environments should be designed or adapted to meet the needs of people. It is important to consult the regulations that apply to your locale before starting housing improvements.

TABLE 5.2
Description and Examples of Regulations Category

Topic	Description	Example
Universal accessibility standards	Universal accessibility means that the environment must be usable by anyone, regardless of their physical or cognitive abilities. International standards, such as the ISO 21542 guidelines (Accessibility and Usability of the Built Environment), and national regulations, such as the Brazilian Inclusion Law (LBI) or the Americans with Disabilities Act (ADA) in the US, establish requirements for accessibility in residential and public buildings	Door widths, ramp slopes, elevator dimensions, installation of grab bars with user-centered design
Ergonomic standards	Ergonomic standards refer to the design of spaces and furniture in a way that minimizes physical effort and facilitates activities of daily living	Ideal height for sinks, countertops, beds and chairs, as well as the proper positioning of cabinets and everyday utensils
Standards for sanitary facilities	Some countries have regulations that indicate the need to adapt these environments to ensure safety and accessibility. Some standards can stipulate the minimum dimensions and equipment required for this space	Shower stalls without unevenness or doors, the provision of grab bars in strategic locations, and the use of water-resistant and non-slip materials
Lighting standards	Poor lighting is one of the factors that most contribute to falls among older adults. Lighting standards recommend the use of brighter and well-distributed lights in circulation areas, such as hallways, stairs, and bathrooms, in addition to the installation of accessible switches or automated systems. Some regulations include the adaptation of natural lighting to reduce shadows and reflections	Bright, well-distributed lighting, motion-activated lighting, accessible light switches, automated lighting systems, glare reduction, staircase lighting, night lights, color temperature consideration

The benefits of following regulations are that these standards will ensure that the environment will be designed or adapted in accordance with the minimum criteria and conditions to become safe. Regulations can help to improve the quality of life, comfort, promoting healthier, independent, and comfortable aging.

5.4 EQUIPMENT

Equipment refers to devices, utensils, and tools designed to improve safety, accessibility, and comfort for residents, described in Table 5.3. Equipment helps to compensate for physical and cognitive limitations common with aging, facilitating daily living activities, preventing accidents, and promoting greater independence. With appropriate equipment it is possible to improve a functional and safe environment for users.

TABLE 5.3
Description and Examples of Equipment Category

Topic	Description	Example
Grab bars	Provide physical support, helping the person to balance and move around more safely	Install in areas with a higher risk of falls, such as bathrooms, hallways, and stairs
Accessible appliances	Appliances are essential to make life easier, especially those with mobility, vision, or hearing difficulties	Simplified controls, large and visible buttons, and automated functions like ovens and stoves with front controls, refrigerators with easy-to-open doors, and front-loading washing machines
Seat bath	Devices for older adults who have difficulty standing for long periods or sitting and getting up on their own during bath	Shower chair with backrest and arms, transfer bench, folding shower seat

The benefits of using equipment are that most of them increase safety, allow greater autonomy, provide comfort, and help to prevent injuries. Installing appropriate equipment is a fundamental strategy to ensure safety because these devices help mitigate the risks associated with aging and provide an environment that facilitates the performance of daily living activities.

5.5 ASSISTIVE TECHNOLOGY

Assistive technologies are a range of devices, products, and systems that help people with physical, sensory, or cognitive disabilities to perform everyday tasks more independently and safely. In the context of housing, these technologies play a fundamental role in improving quality of life, promoting greater independence and comfort within the home. In Table 5.4 are detailed descriptions of this category.

With aging, natural limitations arise related to mobility, vision, hearing, memory, and muscle strength. Assistive technologies come precisely to compensate for these limitations, allowing people to continue to live independently for longer.

TABLE 5.4
Description and Examples of Assistive Technology Category

Topic	Description	Example
Communication devices	For older adults with hearing or visual impairments, assistive technologies can improve communication	Hearing aids with advanced sound adjustment features, telephones with large letters and voice-assisted speakers, such as voice command systems that help seniors control lights, electronic devices, and even make phone calls

TABLE 5.4 *(Continued)*
Description and Examples of Assistive Technology Category

Topic	Description	Example
Monitoring and security systems	These devices can enhance safety and support remote monitoring systems, enabling family members or caregivers to oversee the routine of older adults from a distance	Motion sensors, monitoring cameras, emergency alarm devices (such as panic buttons), fall, smoke, and light sensors
Smart appliances	Household devices equipped with advanced technology that make daily tasks easier, safer, and more efficient. These appliances are often connected to the internet and can be controlled remotely via smartphones or voice-activated systems	Smart refrigerators, stoves, or ovens with automatic shut-off features to prevent accidents; voice-activated lights or thermostats; smart medication dispensers; fall detection systems and smart locks

The benefits of using assistive technologies are to guarantee promotion of independence, increase the sense of safety, prevent accidents, emergencies, and integration with healthcare systems.

5.6 CONSTRUCTION MATERIALS

Construction materials in the context of a housing environment refers to elements used in the construction or renovation of a residence that directly affect the safety, accessibility, and comfort. These materials include, for example, floors, coverings, colors, doors, windows, etc.

Construction materials are essential in creating safe environments, as the physical characteristics of the space, such as texture, color, grip and height, can directly influence the ability to move around and perform daily living activities, as presented in Table 5.5. The correct choice of these materials ensures greater safety and comfort, in addition to preventing accidents.

TABLE 5.5
Description and Examples of Construction Materials Category

Topic	Description	Example
Non-slip floors	Flooring is one of the most critical elements when it comes to environmental safety. To prevent falls, which are the main cause of domestic accidents among older adults, it is essential to use non-slip flooring, especially in wet areas such as kitchens, bathrooms, and utility areas	Textured vinyl flooring, rubber flooring, non-slip ceramic or porcelain tiles, laminate flooring with non-slip finish

(Continued)

TABLE 5.5 *(Contineud)*
Description and Examples of Construction Materials Category

Topic	Description	Example
Wall coverings	Wall coverings play an important role in the safety and comfort	Easy-to-clean materials, such as tiles or washable paints, are essential in areas such as bathrooms and kitchens, where humidity and dirt can be constant
Colors	It is important in both the psychological aspect and the functionality of a space	Use contrast of colors to help users see barriers with more clarity, especially for those who have visual limitations

The choice of flooring, coverings, colors, and other materials has a direct impact on preventing accidents, improving mobility and creating a more welcoming and functional environment. When these materials are thought of in an integrated and planned way, it is possible to transform the home into a space that promotes active and healthy aging, allowing older adults to live with dignity.

5.7 FURNITURE

Furniture includes chairs, beds, sofas, tables, cabinets, shelves, and other elements that must be adapted to the physical and cognitive needs of older adults. Choosing the right furniture can promote greater independence, reduce the risk of accidents, and increase comfort in activities of daily living, as indicated in Table 5.6. Therefore, furniture must be ergonomic, safe, accessible, and adapted to the limitations of mobility and strength that arise with aging.

TABLE 5.6
Description and Examples of Furniture Category

Topic	Description	Example
Appropriate height	The height of furniture is one of the main concerns when adapting the environment for users	Chairs, sofas, and beds, for example, must be at a height that allows the person to sit down and stand up without great difficulty. Furniture that is too low may require extra effort to stand up, while furniture that is too high may be difficult to access
Stable and firm furniture	The stability of furniture is essential to prevent accidents. Furniture that wobbles or is unstable can cause falls or accidents when leaning on it	Armchairs and sofas should have a solid and stable structure, while tables and shelves should be well-fixed and firm

TABLE 5.6 *(Continued)*
Description and Examples of Furniture Category

Topic	Description	Example
Non-slip and comfortable materials	The use of non-slip materials on sofas, chairs and beds helps to prevent slipping, both when sitting and getting up. In addition, it is essential that the furniture offers comfort, with firm cushions that provide good support for the body	Non-slip fabric upholstery, firm, supportive cushions, textured wooden furniture, adjustable recliners with non-slip surfaces
Rounded edges	Furniture with rounded or protected edges reduces the risk of injuries, especially in passageways	Tables, shelves, and chairs with rounded corner

Furniture is fundamental in adapting environments for older adults, being an important factor that influences safety, comfort, and independence within the home. By adapting furniture according to the physical and cognitive needs of the residents, it is possible to create a safe and welcoming environment, where the resident can live with greater autonomy and well-being.

5.8 MAINTENANCE

Maintenance refers to a set of continuous and preventive actions to ensure that living environments are always safe, functional, and adequate to the needs of their residents. Maintenance covers both the structural part of the property, such as repairs and aspects related to the organization, cleaning and preservation of the space, such as the items outlined in Table 5.7. For older adults, this care is essential, as the lack of adequate maintenance can result in unsafe environments that are prone to accidents.

TABLE 5.7
Description and Examples of Maintenance Category

Topic	Description	Example
Structural maintenance and repairs	Refer to the ongoing efforts to ensure that the physical framework of a home remains safe, functional, and accessible	Inspection and repair of physical elements of the house, such as floors, walls, roofs, plumbing, and electrical systems
Regular cleaning	It is an essential part of maintenance. Clean environments promote emotional well-being and reduce the stress caused by clutter	Accumulated dust, dirty floors, or slippery surfaces can increase the risk of respiratory problems, allergies, and falls

(Continued)

TABLE 5.7 *(Continued)*
Description and Examples of Maintenance Category

Topic	Description	Example
Organization	Strategic arrangement and management of furniture, objects, and spaces within the home to ensure safety, easy of movement, and accessibility. A well-organized home environment is essential for preventing falls	Keeping objects in their places, without excess furniture or items that obstruct circulation areas, is essential to ensure the safety of older adults
Repairs	Regular and timely repairs are essential for maintaining the home's structural integrity, preventing accidents	Fixing, restoring, or replacing damaged, worn-out, or malfunctioning elements of the home to ensure a safe, comfortable, and accessible living environment
Maintenance of grab bars and safety equipment regularly	Some items of the house should be inspected to ensure that they are securely installed, providing the necessary support. In addition, safety systems such as alarms and motion sensors should be tested regularly	Checking grab bars, handrails, and other safety equipment installed in the home is vital

Maintenance is an essential aspect in creating safe and functional living environments for older adults. By carrying out frequent repairs, ensuring the cleanliness and organization of the space, and keeping equipment and appliances in good condition, it is possible to prevent accidents, improve comfort, and ensure a better quality of life. Well-maintained and organized environments promote safety and well-being, in addition to reducing the need for emergency and costly interventions in the future.

In this chapter, categories that were developed to facilitate home improvement were detailed to clarify their importance to enlightening aging in place at home for older adults. As mentioned earlier, some of these categories require more time and financial investment for implementation. However, there are adaptations that can be made immediately in the homes, with little or no cost, such as organization and cleaning. It is important to note that these categories will be further explored in the practical approach section.

Section II

Practical Approach

6 Practical Design Considerations Overview

In the following chapters, a practical approach will be taken to present design considerations aimed at enhancing safety for older adults' housing environments. Figure 6.1 serves as a template for how design considerations for each environment will be structured in the subsequent chapters. Each space will feature a detailed visual representation of the classification of its components, integrating textual descriptions, icons, and a color-coded rating system to improve clarity and comprehension.

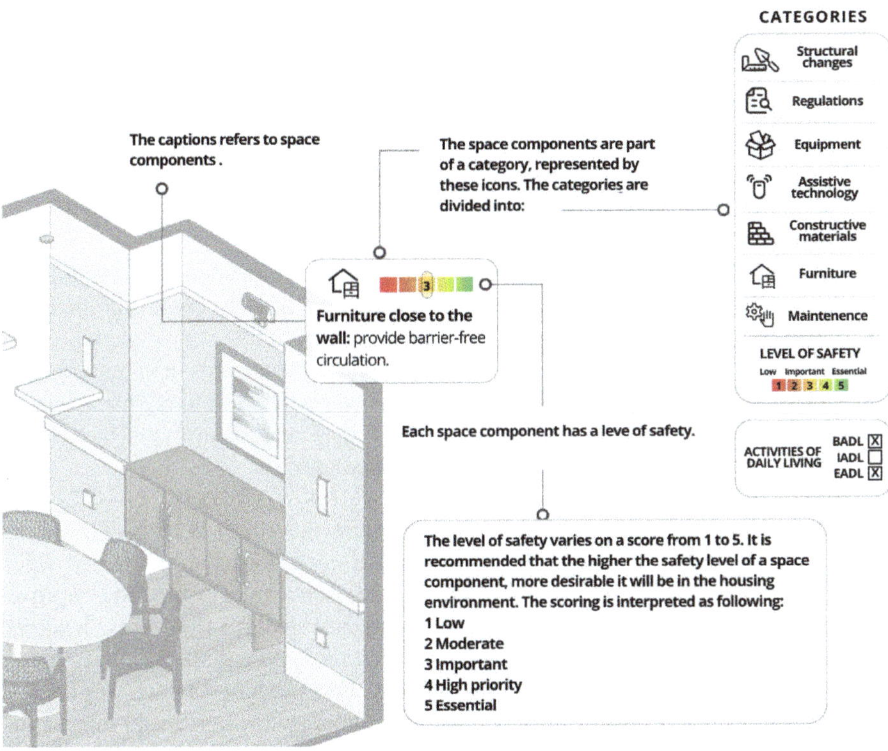

FIGURE 6.1 Guide to interpreting the design considerations for each housing environment based on safety level.

DOI: 10.1201/9781003543701-8

Figure 6.1 represents a series of key elements that can be observed and are essential for understanding the **design considerations** discussed in the following chapters of this book. The icons, text boxes, and color-coded scale provide a multilayered approach to presenting information, combining visual and textual data for clarity. Each **space component** recommended is part of a category and has a safety level. The **categories** are detailed in Chapter 5, divided into structural changes, regulations, equipment, assistive technology, constructive materials, furniture, and maintenance.

The **level of safety** is represented by a combination numerical rating and color code. The numerical rating is from 1 (low) to 5 (essential) and represents the importance of the component, as follows:

- 1—Low safety: the attributes related to this level of safety have minimal impact on safety. It enhances comfort and usability, but their absence does not pose significant risks for users. Additionally, they are not essential for preventing accidents and can be considered optional improvements.
- 2—Moderate safety: this rating makes some contribution to safety but is not critical. It provides a moderate degree of safety benefits and supports a safer environment. Their absence could lead to moderate risks, so they should be prioritized in the long term.
- 3—Important for safety: attributes in this level play key roles in accident prevention and usability, and should be considered in the short term. Its presence in a home environment directly impacts upon safety and usability, and their absence could lead to accidents.
- 4—High safety priority: this rating is strongly recommended for preventing accidents and ensuring safety, and its absence is likely to cause significant risks in the near future.
- 5—Essential for safety: critical for preventing accidents and ensuring usability, and components with this level of safety are absolutely necessary to prevent severe risks and ensure a functional and secure environment. Their absence poses an immediate and critical danger.

The higher the level of safety, the more important the component is. The rating serves to indicate the degree to which each component must be prioritized when designing or adapting a housing environment, and users can prioritize the improvements based on these levels. For example, components rated as 1 (low) are considered less important for safety compared to those rated as 5 (essential). This rating was developed based on a matrix of **severity, urgency, and tendency**, which was applied to each component in housing environments. The color serves as a visual representation and varies to green (5—essential), which indicates that the component should be prioritized to red (1—low) that suggests lower priority. As the number decreases, the importance and safety level of the component also decrease.

In the top right corner of Figure 6.1, the **Categories** are represented with icons, as each space component is associated with a specific category, as introduced in Chapter 5. Below the category panel, the corresponding **activities of daily living** related to the environment being presented are listed, where each environment may support different types of activities, as contextualized in Chapter 2, Section 2.2.

The housing environments presented in the following chapters appear according to the flow of entering a typical home. We start with the front door, followed by the living room, dining room, kitchen, laundry room, bathroom, bedroom, closet, and home office. Finally, design considerations for additional spaces such as the garage and outdoor areas are also provided. These chapters are organized beginning with a general overview of the space, followed by space components followed by design considerations through images (as exemplified in Figure 6.1) along with the practical applications.

7 Front Door

7.1 OVERVIEW OF SPACE

The front door is a significant space for users as they enter or leave the home. It serves as a threshold between the secure interior and the external environment, directly impacting residents' sense of safety, accessibility, and independence. For older adults, the design and functionality of this area should prioritize features that reduce the risk of accidents, ensure ease of access, and enhance comfort. The activities of daily living performed in this space are the basic (e.g., entering and exiting the home safely, locking and unlocking the door, and preparing to go outside) and enhanced (e.g., receiving deliveries or mail, interacting with visitors, and etc.).

7.2 SPACE COMPONENTS

The space components to improve home environment for a safe aging in place will be described according to the level of safety, from minimum to maximum.

For the front door, assistive technologies play a crucial role in improving the accessibility and usability of environments for older adults, especially in the context of their homes. One such technology is an automatic **opening and closing mechanism** for doors, which can significantly enhance convenience and independence. This system allows the door to open automatically when activated, eliminating the need for any physical effort from the user.

Design elements and visual communication can further enhance the living environment for older adults. For example, the entrance door should be designed in a distinctive way that helps the resident easily recognize their home. Such design features contribute to spatial orientation, aiding in memory retention and ensuring the home is easily distinguishable within the neighborhood. Effective visual communication includes clear and legible numbering of the home, positioned in a location where it is easily visible. The font format and size should be chosen for optimal legibility, and the color contrast between the numbers and the background should be carefully considered to ensure maximum visibility for individuals with varying levels of visual acuity.

Benches or other supportive seating are crucial for aiding during the process of entering or exiting the home. However, these pieces of furniture should be carefully considered as they represent an additional element to be incorporated into the space. It is essential to strategically place these benches to avoid creating obstructions that could pose a risk of accidents or hinder movement, ensuring they contribute to the overall accessibility and safety of the environment. **Support tables** can be placed near the door to hold bags and equipment while entering home.

 DOI: 10.1201/9781003543701-9

An **intercom or other communication device** is recommended to be installed between the external and internal environments to facilitate interaction and ensure safety and convenience, particularly for individuals with mobility or hearing impairments. As an example, a ring video doorbell which is a smart home device equipped with a built-in camera, microphone, and speaker. It allows users to see, hear, and communicate with visitors, and enables older adults to identify and interact with people at the front door without the need to physically open it—enhancing both safety and convenience.

Another essential element to consider is the use of **lever-type door handles**. These handles are more accessible and easier to operate, particularly for users who experience difficulties with grip strength. It is also important to ensure that door handles and switches (preferably lever types), and other frequently used items are within easy reach for users.

Artificial lighting is a key feature to improve safety, especially in areas with limited or no natural light as it helps identify physical barriers and obstacles. In addition, during a power outage, **emergency lighting** becomes essential as it ensures safe navigation and access to the home. Incorporating **color contrast** is highly recommended to enhance safety. For example, the entrance door can be painted in a color that contrasts with the surrounding walls, making it more visible and easier to identify. Moreover, a **presence sensor** can be installed to automatically activate the artificial lighting when someone approaches the door. This eliminates the need to put down bags or other objects to turn on the light, ensuring a smooth and safe entry into the home.

The installation of a **ramp** is highly recommended for Front Door, as it provides safer movement, although structural modifications may often be required. Another essential feature to enhance mobility is the installation of **grab bars/handrails**, which guide users safely and offer additional support. To facilitate access, these equipment should be strategically placed, and **steps or uneven surfaces should be avoided whenever possible**.

Given that the entrance door serves as a transition between the external and internal environments, it is crucial to consider the external area, which may become wet during rainy days. The presence of proper **drainage** systems can help prevent water accumulation and minimize the risk of slips.

Additionally, **non-slip flooring** should be used to ensure safe movement within the space. This type of flooring not only provides better grip and friction but also reduces glare, which is common with polished floors. For individuals who may need to look down while walking, this is particularly important, as glare can significantly hinder movement, especially for those with sensitive vision.

If opting to use rugs in the entryway, it is important that the **rug be level with the floor** to avoid creating any tripping hazards. The recommendation is for the rug to be recessed into the floor to minimize the risk of trips and falls.

Other general recommendations are, for example, an **entrance hall as a supportive area** for those entering the home. This space not only provides greater privacy in relation to the other areas of the house but also serves as a functional zone for items such as sideboards, coat racks, and shoe racks—essential accessories for people entering or leaving the home.

Windows with a lower sill are another key element that enhance the front door entrance space. In addition to providing **natural light** and **ventilation**, these windows allow for **better visibility** of the outside, contributing to access control and security by enabling residents to monitor who is entering or leaving the home.

Special attention should be given to the regulations governing the sizing **of architectural elements**. For instance, when designing the access door, it is essential to consider not only the relevant regulations but also the specific needs and mobility challenges of the users. This process ensures that the entrance remains **comfortable and appropriately dimensioned for easy access**.

Additionally, the use of **water-resistant materials** is strongly recommended to minimize the need for frequent maintenance and to prevent hazards related to wear and tear. Choosing durable materials helps maintain the integrity of the finishes and coverings in this area, ensuring long-term safety and functionality.

In summary, the front door area must ensure safety and comfort for older adults within their homes. The integration of assistive technologies demonstrates how thoughtful design can address both functional and sensory limitations. In parallel, design strategies help to promote independence. When designing the front door area, certain considerations must be aligned with the accessibility **standards and regulations** of each country. These regulations often provide important guidelines—for example, the maximum slope allowed for ramps or the required positioning and specifications of handrails. Therefore, it is essential to consult these standards during the design process to ensure compliance and safety. In addition to following national regulations, it is equally important to consider the specific physical and cognitive abilities of the users who will interact with the space. A truly effective and inclusive design goes beyond regulatory requirements by being tailored to the real needs and limitations of its users, especially in residential environments for older adults. By adopting a user-centered approach and implementing practical, evidence-based modifications, the front door space can become a safer, more welcoming threshold—one that supports activities of daily living, encourages independence, and fosters a sense of security for aging in place.

7.3 DESIGN CONSIDERATIONS

Guidelines for the front door design are organized into categories according to safety levels, making it easier to identify and prioritize specific design attributes, as shown in Figure 7.1. Note that all of the elements labeled 4 (high priority) or 5 (essential) are especially important to attend to. The design recommendations presented would help to ensure a level of safety that is in the direction of green, meaning higher safety. Less critical elements (labeled 1 and 2) would also benefit from the design recommendation to increase safety, but could be prioritized to a lesser degree.

Thus for the front door, the most critical elements to address are lighting, presence sensors, drainage, color contrast, ramps, rugs, grab bars, and non-slip floors. The guidelines suggested in Figure 7.1 are just examples—there may be other solutions. But the guidance provides an indicator of the priorities for this space.

The focus of the chapter has been on the front door, assuming that is the most frequently utilized entrance to the home. However, many homes have multiple entry points (e.g., a back door, a side door entry from a garage) that would also have to be scrutinized in a similar fashion to identify safety elements that need to be addressed.

Key Points

- **Non-slip flooring:** install anti-slip surfaces to prevent falls, especially in areas exposed to water or low lighting.
- **Avoid rugs:** rugs should either be avoided or embedded (recessed) into the flooring to eliminate tripping hazards.
- **Accessibility-compliant ramp:** incorporate ramps designed according to each country's accessibility regulations and principles of universal design, ensuring safe and easy access for all users.
- **Drain:** add a floor drain near the entrance to prevent water accumulation during rainy weather, reducing the risk of slipping.
- **Artificial lighting**: include both artificial and emergency lighting to improve visibility and safety, especially at night or during power outages. Use presence sensors for automatic activation.
- **Color contrast:** use contrasting colors between key elements (e.g., door vs. wall, signage vs. background) to aid visibility, particularly for individuals with low vision.

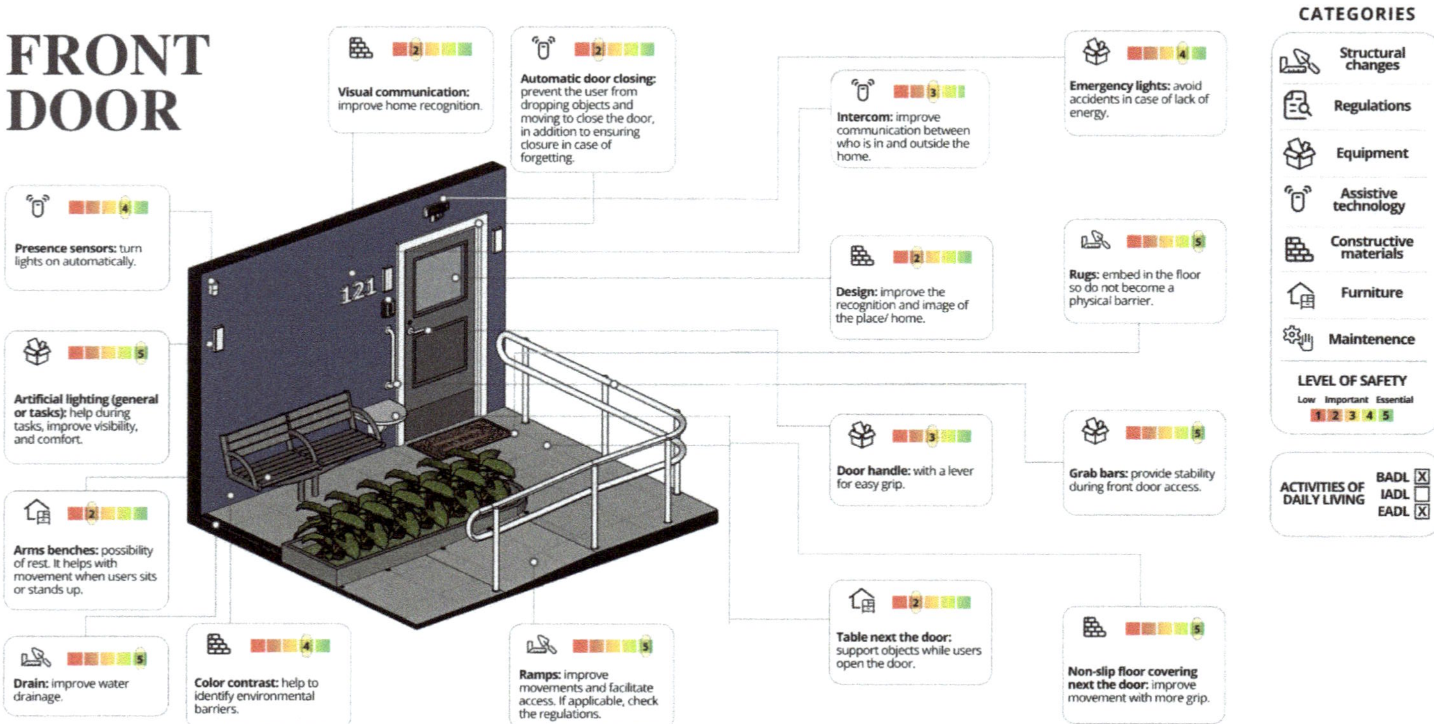

FIGURE 7.1 Design guidelines for front door.

8 Living Room

8.1 OVERVIEW OF SPACE

The space components of the living room are organized in this chapter from the minimum to maximum level of safety.

The living room area often is integrated into the main social environment of the home. From an architectural standpoint, when analyzing the spatial layout of a residence, the living room is usually located near the main entrance (front door). Typically, following the living room in the floor plan, the dining room appears as a complementary social space, reinforcing the function of these environments as areas for gathering and socialization within the household. Activities of daily living performed in this space are basic (e.g., resting or sitting) and enhanced (e.g., hosting visitors or family gatherings or using digital devices or smart technologies for communication or entertainment).

8.2 SPACE COMPONENTS

The living room space components to improve home environment for aging in place safely are organized below according to the level of safety, from minimum to maximum.

The space components to improve home environment for safe aging in place will be described according to the level of safety, from minimum to maximum. **Personalizing the decoration** by incorporating personal items and familiar elements near the entrance fosters emotional attachment to the home environment. This supports identity, memory, and a sense of control—factors that are especially important in aging in place strategies. For **curtains** it is recommended that they be made of flame-retardant fabrics to enhance fire safety. Floor-length curtains are discouraged due to the potential for entanglement or tripping. Simplified designs, such as blinds, are easier to operate and maintain.

Another important characteristic that can be implemented when possible is a **low window** that allows seated users—such as those in wheelchairs or using walkers—to maintain visual contact with the exterior environment. This feature supports orientation, enhances natural surveillance, and reinforces psychological well-being by connecting the individual with their surroundings. When choosing furniture, **armchairs or chairs should have armrests** which will provide leverage for older adults when sitting down or standing up, a movement that becomes more difficult with age due to decreased muscle strength and joint flexibility. These supports help maintain functional independence in daily routines. Furniture with simple, stable forms minimizes the risk of tripping. Avoiding curved or splayed legs in circulation areas reduces visual clutter and physical obstacles.

DOI: 10.1201/9781003543701-10

Concerning assistive technology, an **accessible emergency alarm** ensures that help can be summoned quickly in the event of a fall, medical emergency, or security issue. Its presence promotes peace of mind and encourages older adults to maintain their independence. A **matte wooden flooring** is ideal, as non-glossy wooden floors reduce glare, improving visibility and comfort. Additionally, matte finishes typically offer better slip resistance, making them safer for individuals using canes, walkers, or who are otherwise at risk of falls.

As mentioned in Chapter 7, **backup lighting** that can be activated during power outages is vital for fall prevention, especially for older adults with visual impairments or balance issues. Ensuring visibility during emergencies supports both safety and autonomy. **Motion-activated lighting** assists with nighttime orientation by automatically illuminating pathways and key areas when movement is detected, facilitating safe movement and reducing the risk of trips or falls in low-light conditions. This type of lighting is especially helpful for older adults who may experience disrupted sleep patterns or need to navigate their home during the night without fumbling for switches. By providing hands-free, timely illumination, motion-activated lighting also helps reduce anxiety and promotes greater independence during nighttime activities. Adequate lighting improves visual comfort and reduces shadows and glare. This type of lighting is essential for tasks such as key insertion, mail retrieval, or interacting with visitors—activities that may become challenging with age-related vision decline.

Color contrast schemes play a crucial role in helping older adults with reduced visual acuity identify potential environmental barriers and distinguish between different surfaces such as floor levels, thresholds, and furnishings. Well-designed contrast enhances spatial orientation, supports cognitive mapping, and significantly reduces the risk of missteps and falls.

Smoke sensors are crucial in homes with older residents, who may have slower reaction times or limited mobility. Smoke sensors contribute to passive safety and enable timely evacuation or emergency response. Strategically installed **grab bars** provide essential support for balance and weight transfer during movement. They are especially beneficial when transitioning between standing and sitting positions, helping to reduce the risk of falls—one of the leading causes of injury among older adults. Although grab bars are commonly associated with bathrooms or entryways, they are often overlooked in living room settings. However, considering the amount of time older adults typically spend in the living room and the frequency of transfers between seated and standing positions, these supports should not be disregarded in this space. When thoughtfully integrated, grab bars can enhance safety without compromising the aesthetic quality of the environment—particularly when designed with discreet or decorative elements that blend with the overall interior design.

Other important design strategies include positioning furniture along walls to create wider, unobstructed circulation paths. This spatial approach **minimizes physical barriers**, significantly reducing the risk of falls—especially for individuals who use mobility aids such as walkers or canes. **Clear and accessible pathways** also promote safe, independent movement, which in turn fosters a greater sense of confidence and autonomy within the space.

Certain elements, however, should be avoided in environments such as the living room. Uneven flooring and loose rugs are common contributors to trips and falls and should be eliminated whenever possible. That said, the use of rugs may still be preferred for cultural or aesthetic reasons, as they can contribute to a sense of warmth and comfort. In such cases, rugs should be recessed into the floor so that their surface is flush with the surrounding flooring. This requires structural modifications but provides a much safer solution. By implementing safety measures such as avoiding uneven surfaces and securing rugs properly, a minimum standard of safety can be maintained. Additionally, when selecting flooring materials, it is advisable to choose those with sound-absorbing properties to help minimize ambient noise and enhance acoustic comfort within the space.

Designing the living room for aging in place requires a thoughtful balance between functionality, safety, and comfort. As a central area for daily activities and social interaction, the living room should be adapted to meet the physical, cognitive, and sensory needs of older adults. Key strategies include ensuring unobstructed circulation paths, using non-slip and low-glare flooring, optimizing lighting with motion sensors and backup systems, and incorporating high-contrast color schemes to enhance visibility and orientation. Integrating grab bars, fire safety devices, and accessible furniture promotes independence and reduces the risk of injury. Moreover, attention to personal elements—such as meaningful decor and familiar objects—helps foster a strong emotional connection to the space. By combining universal design principles with specific safety measures, the living room can be transformed into an inclusive environment that supports autonomy, well-being, and quality of life as individuals age at home.

For living room environments, both general and specific regulations may apply (it is important to consult the standards relevant to each country). In general, beyond focusing on the users' physical and cognitive needs and abilities, the space should be designed with dimensions (width × length) that are compatible with the intended functions. Circulation areas, in addition to being free of barriers, must provide sufficient width to allow for safe movement—some countries recommend a minimum of 80 to 120 cm (approximately 32 to 48 inches). Other regulations may also apply to the dimensions of openings (such as doors and windows), as well as the height and placement of switches and electrical outlets. Other standards that can be consulted to complement the information in the guidelines include: Thermal and Environmental Comfort Standards, Acoustic Standards, Accessible Signage and Communication (when applicable), Fire Safety and Prevention Standards, and Standards for Assistive Technology and Home Automation.

8.3 DESIGN CONSIDERATIONS

Guidelines for the living room are organized into categories according to safety levels, making it easier to identify and prioritize specific design attributes, as shown in Figure 8.1.

Key Points

- **Artificial lighting**: including emergency backup lighting and motion-activated night lighting, to ensure safety and comfort during low-light conditions or power outages.
- **Color contrast:** improve visibility and spatial orientation, helping to distinguish surfaces and reduce fall risks.
- **Ergonomic chairs and armchairs with armrests:** support safe sitting and standing movements, enhancing functional independence.
- **Grab bars:** to aid balance and weight transfer, particularly during transitions between sitting and standing.
- **Smoke detectors:** to provide early warning and enhance passive safety for timely evacuation or emergency response.

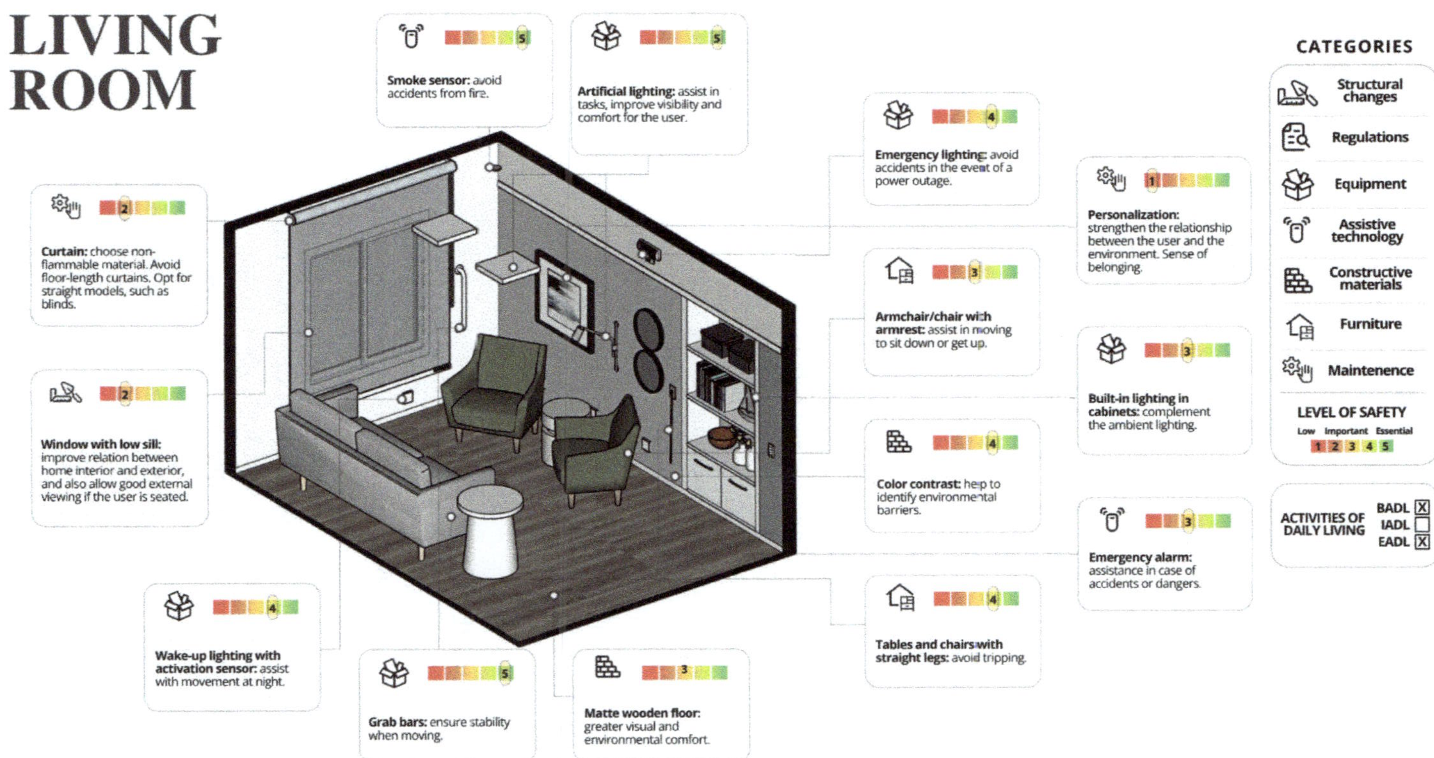

FIGURE 8.1 Design guidelines for the living room.

9 Dining Room

9.1 OVERVIEW OF SPACE

The space components of the dining room are organized in this chapter from the minimum to maximum level of safety.

Designing the dining room means prioritizing accessibility, comfort, and safety. This includes selecting ergonomic furniture, ensuring adequate lighting, and providing clear circulation pathways for mobility aids and other characteristics. The dining room generally serves a complementary role to both the living room and kitchen and is often integrated into the broader social area of the home. It functions as a central space for shared meals, celebrations, and everyday interactions, fostering social connection and family cohesion. Whether designed as part of an open-plan layout or as a more defined, separate room, the dining room enhances both the spatial flow and functionality of the home.

For older adults, the dining room takes on additional significance beyond mealtime—it becomes a vital setting for maintaining routines, participating in social life, and reinforcing a sense of purpose and belonging. The act of sitting together for meals can support nutritional health and emotional well-being, especially for those at risk of isolation. Activities of daily living (ADLs) carried out in the dining room include basic tasks (e.g., sitting at the table, eating meals, drinking fluids, or taking medication) and enhanced (e.g., hosting visitors for special occasions, participating in family meals with social interaction, or using the space for leisure pursuits such as reading the newspaper, playing board games, organizing mail, or engaging in light crafts and hobbies—especially when the dining area serves multiple functions throughout the day).

9.2 SPACE COMPONENTS

Many of the safety and comfort features for the dining room are also mentioned in the living room chapter, as both spaces serve essential roles in activities of daily living of older adults. These environments are frequently used for social interaction, relaxation, and various everyday activities, making it critical that they are designed with attention to accessibility, safety, and emotional well-being. The following space components focus on the dining room, highlighting design strategies and environmental adaptations that promote independence and reduce risks—many of which can be mirrored or adapted for use in living areas as well. The components of the dining room environment are presented progressively, starting from those associated with a lower level of safety and moving toward those that offer higher levels of safety.

Encouraging a sense of identity, comfort, and belonging is important in every housing space. Various **personalized elements** can support cognitive orientation and reinforce the user's emotional bond with their living space. Window treatments

DOI: 10.1201/9781003543701-11

such as **curtains** should be made of non-flammable materials and designed to avoid contact with the floor. Blinds are easier to manage, safer, and less likely to cause tripping. Also, it is important to consider having **windows with low sills,** which enable seated users to have a clear view of the outdoors, strengthening the connection between interior and exterior environments, and contributes to sensory stimulation, orientation, and mental well-being.

Furniture positioned close to the wall facilitates clear circulation paths, which is especially important for users with limited mobility or those using assistive devices. This layout minimizes obstructions and allows for easier navigation. For flooring materials, it is recommended that they have sound absorption properties in order to minimize possible noise arising from the use of these spaces. For flooring, **wood** is the recommended covering, as long as it has a matte finish. Regarding furniture, armchairs or chairs with armrests are recommended for supporting safe transitions between sitting and standing. Armrests provide stability, reduce physical effort, and help maintain balance. Straight legs for tables and chairs is one kind of characteristic that promotes safety by reducing tripping hazards. Simple leg designs are less likely to interfere with walking aids or foot placement.

Artificial lighting always ensures adequate illumination for everyday tasks, reducing visual strain and enhancing spatial perception. It also contributes to a sense of comfort and security. **Emergency lighting** is another important feature that provides visibility during power outages, helping to prevent accidents and disorientation in critical situations and specially when lighting can be **activated automatically** in low-light conditions, supporting nighttime mobility and minimizing the risk of falls when getting out of bed. For enhancing the ability to distinguish between furniture, floors, and other environmental elements, **color contrast** is especially beneficial for older adults with visual impairments, supporting safer navigation.

Grab bars installed near seating or circulation areas provide essential support for movement and balance, significantly lowering the risk of falls. Assistive technologies such as **smoke sensors** offer early detection of fire-related incidents, ensuring prompt response and enhancing overall safety, particularly in settings where reaction time may be delayed.

Other general recommendations include avoiding the use of rugs and carpets, which can pose tripping hazards, and selecting furniture that is lightweight and easy to move, allowing for greater flexibility and adaptability within the space. An effective strategy when planning the layout is to ensure a barrier-free circulation area, facilitating safe and unobstructed movement for all users, particularly those with mobility limitations.

The dining room is an important space at home and supports both the physical and emotional well-being of older adults due to the fact that it is a place where it is commonly shared with others. It encourages social interaction and reinforces a sense of belonging and participation in daily life. When designing, aspects like accessibility, safety, and comfort must be taken into account to contribute to users' independence and improve the quality of life. When tailored to meet the evolving needs of older adults, the dining room becomes a meaningful, functional, and inclusive space that promotes aging in place with dignity and engagement.

As commented before in the Living Room, for the Dining Room it is also important to focus on the users' physical and cognitive needs and abilities, the space should be designed with dimensions (width × length) that are compatible with the intended functions. Circulation areas, in addition to being free of barriers, must provide sufficient width to allow for safe movement—the standards of some countries recommend a minimum of 80 to 120 cm (approximately 32 to 48 inches). Other regulations may also apply to the dimensions of openings (such as doors and windows), as well as the height and placement of switches and electrical outlets. Always consult the relevant regulations before adapting, designing, constructing, or renovating any space.

9.3 DESIGN CONSIDERATIONS

Guidelines for the dining room are organized into categories according to safety levels, making it easier to identify and prioritize specific design attributes, as shown in Figure 9.1.

Note that there are themes across the living room and the dining room, such as the need for grab bars, the flooring, the placement of furniture, and the lighting. These themes will recur as we move through different areas of the home.

Key Points

- **Artificial lighting**: ensures adequate illumination for everyday tasks, reducing visual strain and enhancing spatial perception and comfort. Emergency and nighttime (wake-up) lighting is equally important for providing automatic illumination during power outages or low-light conditions, supporting safe mobility and reducing fall risk, especially at night.
- **Color contrast**: improves the ability of older adults with visual impairments to distinguish furniture, floors, and other elements, aiding safer navigation within the space.
- **Grab bars**: strategically installed near seating or circulation areas to provide support for movement and balance, significantly lowering the risk of falls.
- **Tables and chairs with straight legs**: furniture with simple, straight legs minimizes tripping hazards and interference with mobility aids, enhancing safety and ease of movement.
- **Smoke sensor**: early detection of fire hazards ensures prompt response, improving overall safety for occupants, particularly where reaction times may be slower.

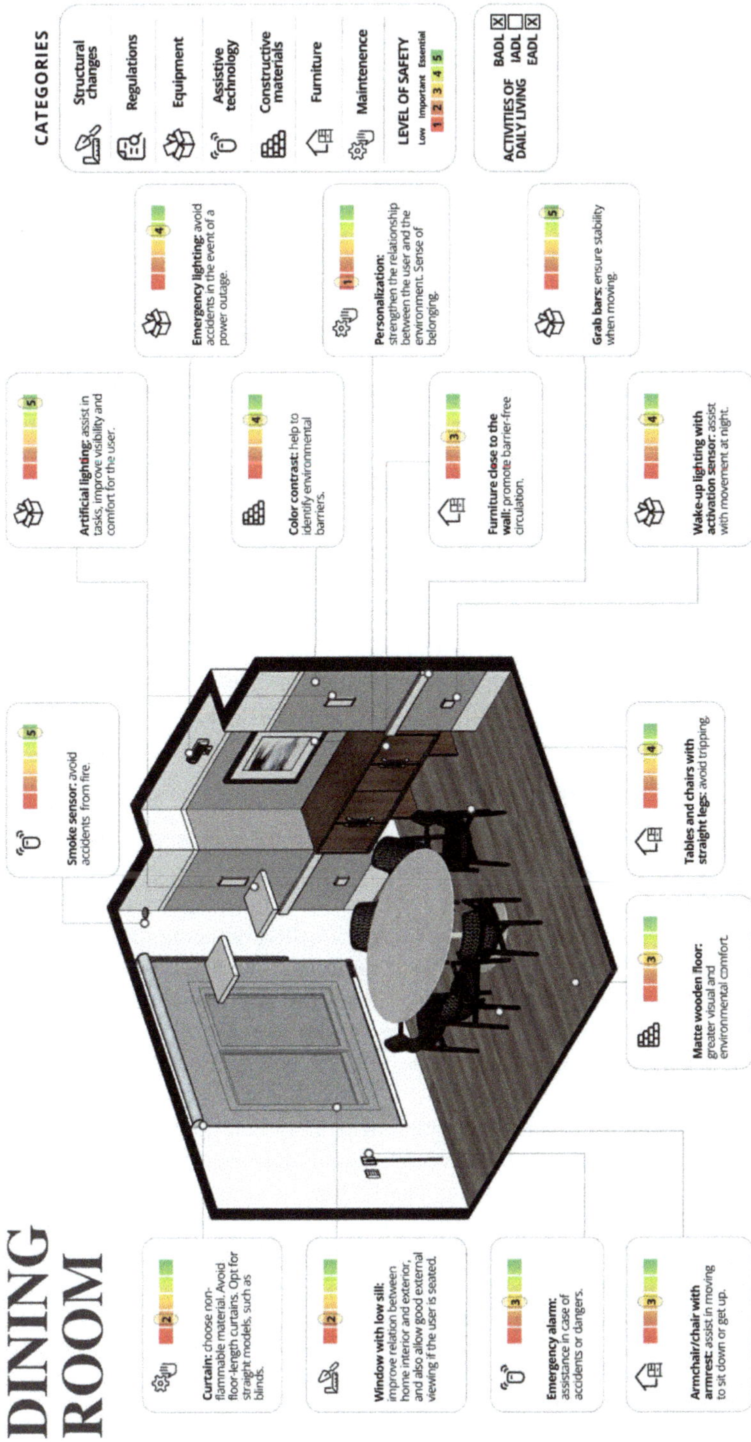

FIGURE 9.1 Design guidelines for the dining room.

10 Kitchen

10.1 OVERVIEW OF SPACE

The space components to improve the kitchen for aging in place safely are organized below from minimum to maximum level of safety.

This is an important space in the home of older adults, as it is where they often spend a significant amount of time engaging in essential daily activities. These include preparing meals, eating, and socializing with family members or visitors. Routine tasks such as accessing the refrigerator, using cabinets and drawers, handling food, operating the stove, oven, or microwave, and washing and storing dishes all require various levels of physical and cognitive effort. Although these activities may appear simple and automatic for most people, they can become challenging for individuals with motor, sensory, or cognitive impairments. For this reason, the kitchen environment must be carefully designed to match the user's abilities, ensuring it is both accessible and safe for daily use. In this space, older adults carry out a range of activities of daily living (ADLs), including basic (e.g., eating meals, drinking fluids, and taking medications), instrumental (e.g., preparing meals, setting the table, and cleaning up), and enhanced (e.g., social interactions, hosting family gatherings, playing games, or enjoying leisure activities with guests).

10.2 SPACE COMPONENTS

For the kitchen, a variety of design recommendations are necessary to improve the use of the space with independence, autonomy, and safety. Using, for example, a **socle in masonry** under sink cabinet is essential for protecting the furniture from water damage. This prevents direct contact with moisture, reducing the risk of swelling, warping, and deterioration, especially in materials like MDF (medium-density fiberboard) or wood. To increase durability, elevating the cabinet makes cleaning easier by preventing dirt buildup and ensuring a more seamless finish with the floor. This simple yet effective design enhances both the longevity and hygiene of the kitchen space.

When selecting **faucets**, choosing models with easy-to-grip controls, preferably **with lever handles** and clear hot and cold-water indicators, offer better usability. Additionally, **thermostatic devices** that visually display water temperature are available on the market. These are easy to install, require no structural modifications, and provide an extra layer of safety by helping prevent burns. Beyond fixtures, heat- and **water-resistant materials** should be prioritized for countertops, cabinet finishes, and flooring, ensuring durability, ease of maintenance, and enhanced safety in the kitchen environment.

Regarding specific design guidelines, it is important to highlight the importance of selecting appropriate kitchen equipment, such as the dishwasher. Traditional models

DOI: 10.1201/9781003543701-12

typically feature a front-opening design, which may require excessive bending and strain. A more functional alternative, especially for older adults, is a **drawer-style dishwasher**, as it allows for easier loading and unloading with minimal effort, improving both accessibility and usability. These appliances have a higher cost in relation to the standard models found in people's homes, but when considering a higher level of safety, the financial investment may also end up being higher in some cases.

When considering furniture, some hinges and slides with dampers and models make opening cabinets easier. Also, if there are **overhead cabinets**, which would not be recommended, one possibility would be to use **glass doors** to make it easier for the user to see what is inside. For the stove, the recommendation is an **induction stove**, which, although more expensive, has greater benefits than a gas stove which involves open flames and the risk of leaks or burns. Induction technology heats only the cookware using electromagnetism, keeping the surface cool and safe to touch, but only certain cookware will work with it. Another alternative would be the use of electric cooktops. While they are a safer option compared to gas stoves, they can still retain heat on the surface after use. Induction cooktops, however, offer greater safety, faster cooking, precise temperature control, and easy cleaning, making them the most suitable and secure option for aging-friendly kitchens.

Users with cognitive impairments may forget to place food in the oven or on the stove, or may leave appliances on unintentionally. To reduce the risk of accidents, **safety sensors** such as **reminder alarms and smart timers** can be installed. These devices help prompt the user to check the food, turn off appliances, or complete cooking tasks—supporting memory and promoting safer, more independent kitchen use. In addition, the position of the household appliances such as stoves and washing machines require specific water, sewage, and gas installations, but can be installed in other places without major changes. In the case of **refrigerators**, depending on the model, movement can be made easier. Preference should be given to **inverse models** (with the freezer at the bottom and the refrigerator on top) or **side-by-side models**, as they are easier to use, and the position of these items must be functional for the performance of the activity.

Key considerations for **built-in lighting in cabinets** is another strategy that serves as a complement to the artificial lighting of the room. Often, when using the worktop, overhead cabinets or the person themselves can cast shadows and make the task more difficult. Integrated cabinet lighting enhances task visibility and provides supplementary illumination alongside the general lighting of the space. Additionally, it is crucial to ensure the presence of a **clearly visible emergency contact** and an easily accessible **emergency alarm** to improve safety in case of accidents. An emergency alarm is a crucial safety feature in the kitchen for older adults. It should be installed within easy reach—ideally near high-risk areas such as the stove, sink, or food preparation surfaces—to allow immediate assistance in case of a fall, burn, or sudden health event.

When selecting furniture, **stools, armchairs, and chairs should have armrests** to assist individuals with sitting down and standing up. **Color contrast** is another feature that can be implemented to help identify barriers. Therefore, it is recommended that floors, walls, and furniture have contrasting colors. For example, an environment that is all the same color, with white floors, walls, and furniture, should be avoided.

Natural lighting is another feature that favors both the entry of light and ventilation. If it is not possible to install a window, at least install **exhaust ventilation** to improve the quality of the air in the internal environment. Regarding **artificial lighting**, especially in areas with limited or no natural light, it is important to help identify physical barriers and obstacles. **Emergency lighting** helps users find their way around and avoid accidents in the event of a power outage; artificial lighting that is positioned and sufficient for carrying out tasks.

Drawers are generally recommended over traditional cabinets, as cabinets often require more bending, reaching, and physical effort to access internal shelves. **Drawers with loop-style pulls** are also preferred, as they are easier to operate—particularly for older adults who may experience arthritis or osteoarthritis in their hands. If there is loose furniture such as **chairs or stools** in the environment, it is important that they have **straight, fixed legs** and are easy to move. The use of rugs should also be avoided, as in addition to accumulating dirt, their thickness can become dangerous. **Non-slip flooring** should be used to ensure safe movement within the kitchen. This type of flooring not only provides better grip and friction but also reduces glare, which is common with polished floors. **Smoke and gas detectors** in the kitchen, especially when used by older adults, provide early warnings of fire hazards and gas leaks, significantly reducing the risk of accidents. Older adults may have slower reaction times or sensory impairments, making it crucial to have an automated alert system that ensures a quick response. Installing audible and visual alarms enhances safety by notifying residents and any caregivers in case of danger. For optimal protection, detectors should be strategically placed near cooking appliances and gas sources, regularly maintained, and equipped with battery backup to function during power outages.

Other strategies that can be easily and cost-effectively implemented without requiring structural modifications include **avoiding the storage of chemical or cleaning products in kitchen cabinets**. When it comes to curtains, if they cannot be eliminated or replaced with blinds, it is essential to choose non-flammable materials for safety. Additionally, careful attention should be given to ensure that **electrical cords are hidden to avoid creating physical barriers** that could impede movement. Placing **furniture close to walls** is another effective way to clear pathways, though in a kitchen, where appliances are essential, a carefully planned layout is crucial to ensure safe and unobstructed movement.

It is important considering **user-centered design** such as a person's reach envelope (i.e., area that can be easily interacted with) that should be considered when specifying the dimensions of kitchen furniture and equipment. Furthermore, in case of tall or overhead cabinets, it is worth noting that to ensure the safety of a person in a room, risky behaviors should be avoided. The presence of a cabinet may cause the older adults to want to access it and climb a stepladder or even use a chair. **Equipment** such as a microwave and other **portable appliances** should be in an **easily accessible** location, within the user's reach, as well as the other appliances in this room.

To improve safety in the kitchen environment, it is also necessary to implement features such as **layout flexibility**, ensuring that the space can be adjusted according to the user's specific needs. The location of this space in relation to the other areas of the house is an important characteristic to take into account. Positioning this room close to the dining room, for example, makes it easier to use the kitchen for meal preparation and serving, while also preventing the person from having to walk long distances carrying objects in their hands.

Simplifying buttons is another aspect for consideration, as many devices have panels with a series of controls, which can cause confusion and stress for those who use them. Investing in devices with this simplification contributes to more efficient use of the device. It is possible to add voice assistants to turn on, turn off, or even program certain devices. For example, remote controls designed for accessibility often feature large, clearly labeled buttons that are easy to see and press. They typically have simple layouts, focusing on essential functions such as power, volume, channel, and input, without the clutter of rarely used buttons. This streamlined design minimizes confusion and enhances ease of use. It is important to note that assistive technology should only be included if the user is familiar with its use. Otherwise, it would not be recommended.

Other criteria to consider is size, so that the space has sufficient measurements to accommodate the activities, users, and equipment. For the kitchen environment, there are some important strategies that can be implemented, such as replacing some types of appliances. Additionally, installing support bars near workstations—such as beside the sink, stove, or countertop—offers older adults essential stability when cooking, cleaning, or moving between tasks.

Designing a kitchen that is accessible, functional, and safe is essential for supporting older adults in maintaining their independence, autonomy, and well-being at home. Through thoughtful design considerations, the kitchen can be transformed into a supportive environment that adapts to the physical and cognitive needs of aging users. A well-designed kitchen contributes not only to daily functioning but also to quality of life, reinforcing a sense of purpose, self-sufficiency, and connection to others.

10.3 DESIGN CONSIDERATIONS

Guidelines for the kitchen are organized into categories according to safety levels, making it easier to identify and prioritize specific design attributes, as shown in Figure 10.1.

Key Points

- **Color contrast**: use contrasting colors for floors, walls, cabinets, and furniture to improve visual perception and help identify barriers, especially for users with visual impairments.
- **Smoke and gas detectors**: install smoke and gas sensors near cooking appliances and gas sources. These should include both audible and visual alarms and be equipped with battery backup to ensure functionality during power outages.

- **Drawer with loop-style pulls**: prefer drawers over traditional cabinets for easier access. Opt for models with loop-style pulls, which are easier to grip.
- **Non-slip flooring**: choose flooring materials with anti-slip properties to reduce fall risks. Avoid glossy finishes and rugs that may cause tripping or sliding.
- **Furniture with straight legs**: select tables, chairs, and stools with straight, fixed legs to minimize tripping hazards and ensure stability. Armrests are also recommended to aid sitting and standing.
- **Artificial and emergency lighting**: ensure sufficient, well-positioned artificial lighting for task visibility. Install emergency lighting systems that activate automatically during power outages to support navigation and reduce disorientation or accidents.
- **Permanent ventilation**: incorporate natural ventilation through windows or ensure mechanical exhaust systems are in place to maintain air quality and remove cooking odors and moisture.

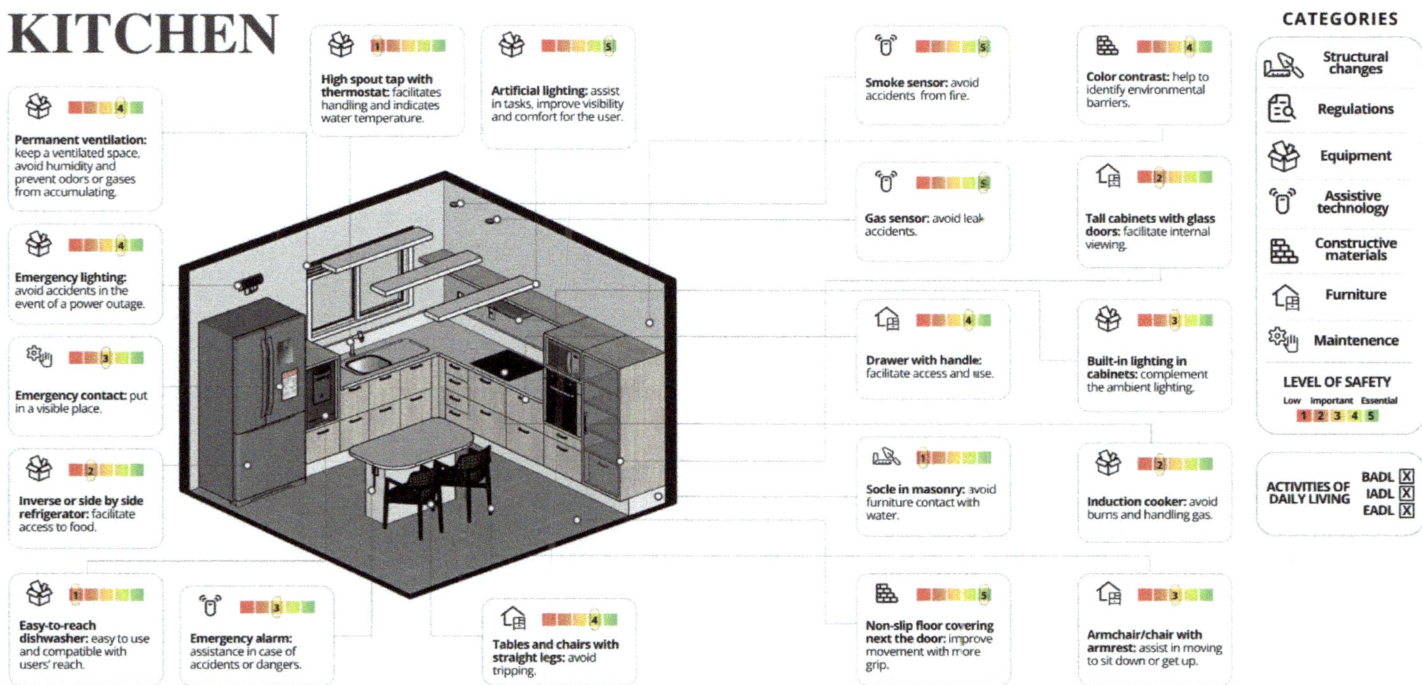

FIGURE 10.1 Design guidelines for the kitchen.

11 Laundry Room

11.1 OVERVIEW OF SPACE

The laundry room space components for improving the home environment to support safe aging in place are described according to the level of safety, from minimum to maximum.

The laundry room is a typically small and compact space in many homes. In some cases, it is integrated into other areas, such as the kitchen or bathroom. Depending on the cultural context, country, or type of housing, these spaces may either not exist at all or be very limited in size. Ideally, there would be a designated room in the house exclusively for laundry tasks, but this is not always feasible. The activity of washing clothes requires effort from the user, as they need to move around to load and unload the washer or dryer. Additionally, hanging clothes involves movements that demand good balance and coordination. In many homes, laundry rooms also serve as storage areas for products and food, so it is crucial that the cabinets are easily accessible. Even when a dedicated laundry room is not possible, it is important to identify and incorporate key features that can improve the functionality of the space, even on a smaller scale. Prioritizing accessibility, safety, and efficient layout can make a significant difference in how the space is used. The activities of daily living performed in this space are instrumental (e.g., loading and unloading the washing machine or dryer, sorting clothes by color or fabric type, folding and organizing clean laundry) and enhanced (e.g., labeling storage bins or containers for better organization, engaging in tasks such as sewing buttons or repairing clothing).

11.2 SPACE COMPONENTS

The first recommendation is to build a **socle in masonry** so that the machines are positioned in a way that is compatible with the users' reach. The position of household appliances and other equipment should be aligned with the activities performed and, therefore, are part of the study of the environment's layout. Additionally, this type of support prevents furniture from coming into contact with water, which helps preserve its durability and structural integrity. The same recommendation was also made for the kitchen environment.

Considering specific recommendations, it is important to highlight that when selecting **faucets** such as those in the kitchen, it is essential to choose models with easy-to-grip controls, preferably **with lever handles** and clear hot- and cold-water indicators for better usability. Additionally, **thermostatic devices** that visually display water temperature are available on the market. In this space, if there is a clothesline for hanging clothes, it is important to choose a model that is easily accessible, ensuring that users can use it without difficulty. The **clothesline** should be positioned

DOI: 10.1201/9781003543701-13

in a way that makes handling easy, allowing the user to operate it without excessive effort or risk of accidents.

Preventing accidents in the laundry room is critical. **Natural lighting** is a feature that provides both illumination and ventilation. If it is not possible to install a window, at least install **exhaust ventilation** to improve the quality of the air in the internal environment. **Artificial lighting** can also improve safety, especially in areas with limited or no natural light, as it helps identify physical barriers and obstacles. **Emergency lighting** is essential because it provides illumination during power outages or emergencies, ensuring that residents can navigate safely in low or no light conditions. It helps prevent accidents, such as falls or collisions, by ensuring that paths, stairways, and exits are clearly visible. **Color contrast** is another feature that can be implemented to help identify barriers. It is recommended that floors, walls, and furniture have contrasting colors. **Drawers** are recommended over cabinets, which require more movement and effort to access the internal shelving area. For drawers as well as cabinets, **loop-style pulls**, as they are easier to use, especially for older adults who may have arthritis or osteoarthritis in their hands.

In a laundry room, especially because there are washing machines and dryers, it is important to install a drain in case of water leaks or overflows. The presence of proper **drainage** systems can help prevent water accumulation and minimize the risk of slips. Another essential feature to enhance mobility is the installation of **grab bars**, which guide users safely and offer additional support. **Non-slip flooring** should be used to ensure safe movement within the space. This type of flooring not only provides better grip and friction but also reduces glare, which is common with polished floors. For individuals who may need to look down while walking, this is particularly important, as glare can significantly hinder movement, especially for those with sensitive vision. When these design safeguards fail and accidents occur, it is important, when possible, to install an **emergency alarm**. **Smoke and gas detectors** provide early warnings of fire hazards and gas leaks, significantly reducing the risk of harm when accidents occur.

General recommendations for this space should consider **avoiding uneven areas**. The **machines**, whether for washing or drying clothes, should be easily **accessible**, centered on the person who will use them. **Smaller coverings** are recommended because they have greater adhesion to ensure safe movement, especially in environments that tend to be humid. **Furniture close to the wall** that allows for freer movement are necessary for the medium level of safety, and the position of equipment and appliances should be part of the layout study and their correlation with the tasks. **Simplifying the buttons** to operate machines, for example, is another factor to be considered. As for the coverings and materials, it is recommended to use options that are **easy to maintain and water-resistant**, such as ceramic tiles, vinyl flooring, quartz countertops, stainless steel, and high-pressure laminates.

Designing a safe and efficient laundry room is essential to support the independence and well-being of older adults. While often a compact or secondary space, the laundry room requires careful attention to layout, reachability, and safety due to the physical demands and potential hazards involved in laundry tasks. All elements from furniture to appliance layout should align with the user's abilities and daily routines.

By addressing these considerations thoughtfully, even small or integrated laundry areas can be transformed into functional, secure, and supportive environments for aging in place.

11.3 DESIGN CONSIDERATIONS

Guidelines for the laundry room are organized into categories according to safety levels, making it easier to identify and prioritize specific design attributes, as shown in Figure 11.1.

Key Points

- **Smoke and gas detectors**: install smoke and gas detectors to provide early warnings of potential hazards, enhancing safety for users with reduced sensory perception or slower reaction times.
- **Permanent ventilation**: ensure continuous air circulation through windows or exhaust systems to reduce humidity, improve air quality, and prevent the buildup of gases or odors.
- **Grab bars**: include strategically placed grab bars to assist with balance and movement, especially when bending, reaching, or performing tasks that require physical effort.
- **Drawer with loop-style pulls**: prefer drawers over traditional cabinets to reduce physical strain. Use loop-style pulls that are easier to grip.
- **Floor drain**: incorporate a well-placed floor drain to prevent water accumulation in case of leaks or spills, reducing the risk of slips and facilitating cleaning.
- **Non-slip flooring**: choose anti-slip floor coverings that provide secure footing and reduce glare, particularly in humid environments, to prevent falls.
- **Color contrast**: use contrasting colors between walls, floors, and furniture to visually differentiate surfaces and enhance spatial orientation, especially for users with visual impairments.
- **Artificial and emergency lighting**: ensure bright, well-distributed artificial lighting for everyday use, and include emergency lighting systems to provide visibility and safety during power outages.

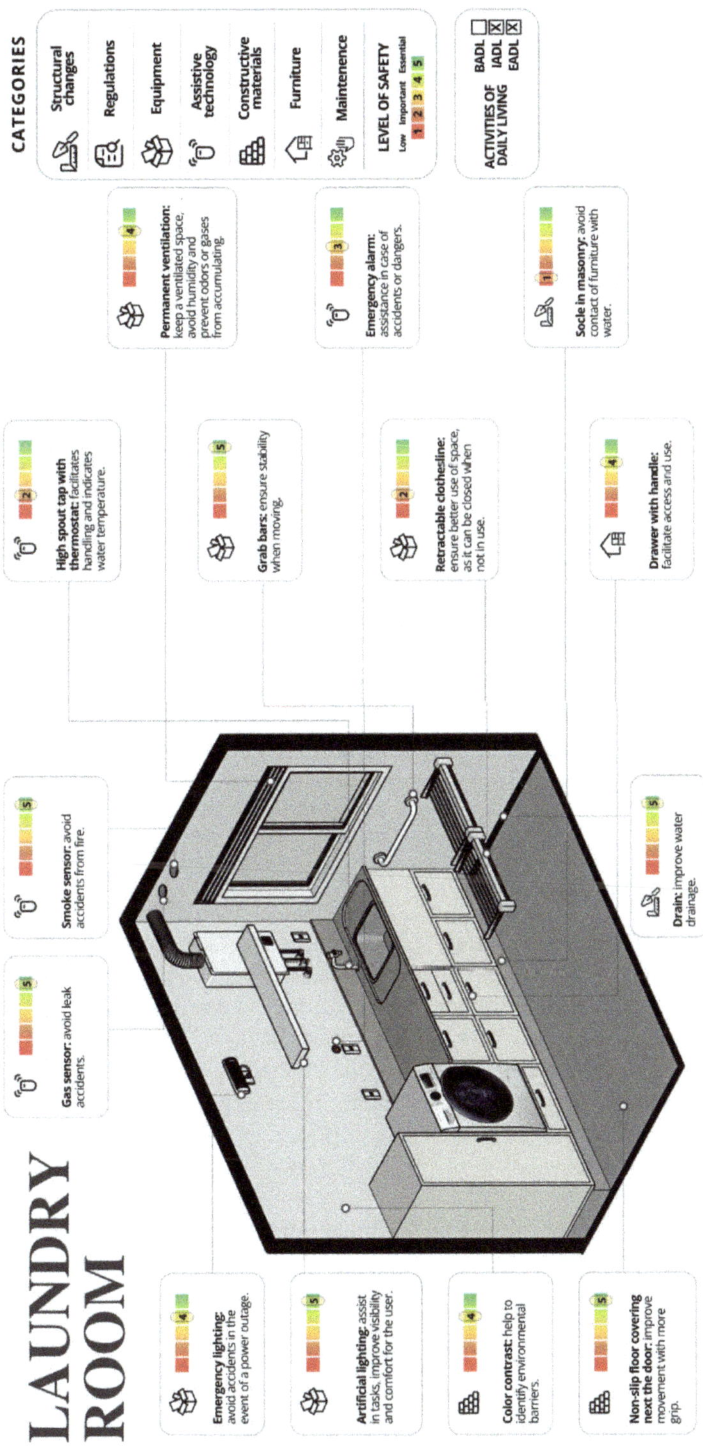

FIGURE 11.1 Design guidelines for the laundry room.

12 Bathroom

12.1 OVERVIEW OF SPACE

The space components to improve the home bathroom environment for a safe aging in place will be described according to the level of safety, from minimum to maximum.

The bathroom is a critical space in the home that requires special attention due to the complexity and physical demands of the activities performed within it. Importantly, numerous studies identify the bathroom as one of the most hazardous areas in the home, especially for older adults. Wet and slippery surfaces, confined spaces, and the need to transfer between positions all contribute to a high risk of falls and injuries, which can result in serious health complications and loss of independence. Given these risks, it is essential to incorporate accessible design features and preventive safety measures so that users can perform daily tasks with greater autonomy, comfort, and safety. Bathrooms are typically one of the smallest rooms in a house, and their reduced size can significantly impact the user's ability to move safely and efficiently, particularly for older adults or individuals with physical limitations. This environment is used for essential basic activities of daily living (e.g., bathing, showering, toileting, grooming, washing hands and face, brushing teeth, dressing or undressing). These activities demand a high level of balance, coordination, flexibility, and sometimes sustained standing or bending. For older adults with reduced strength, mobility, or sensory perception, these actions can become difficult and risky.

12.2 SPACE COMPONENTS

To achieve a minimum level of safety in the bathroom it is recommended to build a **socle in masonry** for furniture mounted to prevent direct contact with water, which not only protects against humidity-related deterioration but also enhances hygiene and safety by reducing the risk of mold or slipping hazards. This solution is consistent with the recommendation also made for the kitchen. In addition, by constructing a base it is possible to adjust the height of the furniture to ensure it is within the user's reach—neither too high nor too low. This contributes to greater comfort, accessibility, and independence, especially for older adults with limited mobility or range of motion.

An anti-fog mirror ensures clear visibility after hot showers without requiring users to wipe the surface, reducing physical effort and avoiding potential slipping caused by condensation. **Faucets** with a **high spout and built-in thermostat** improves accessibility and allows the user to monitor water temperature easily, preventing burns and simplifying the handling of water for hygiene tasks. A **flexible shower head** allows for seated bathing and easier rinsing, while the integrated thermostat prevents scalding and supports safe, independent use of the shower.

 DOI: 10.1201/9781003543701-14

Related to assistive technologies, an **intercom** system facilitates communication with others inside the home, which is essential for emergency situations or regular assistance. Installed within easy reach, the **emergency alarm** allows older adults to call for help in case of accidents such as falls, burns, or sudden health issues. It should be clearly visible and accompanied by an emergency contact number and phone, placed in a prominent location to ensure a prompt response. Backup **lighting systems** activate during a power outage, preventing disorientation and reducing the likelihood of accidents, especially at night or during storms. **Continuous ventilation** helps control humidity, remove odors, and avoid gas accumulation, supporting both health and comfort and can be installed near or beside the window. If the bathroom cannot have a window due to its location within the home, it is essential to install a **mechanical exhaust system**. Proper ventilation is crucial to reduce humidity, prevent mold growth, and maintain air quality, especially in environments frequently exposed to moisture.

Instead of traditional glass doors or shower curtains, it is recommended to install a **masonry half-wall combined with a fixed glass panel.** This design effectively contains water splashes while maintaining an open, unobstructed entryway, making it safer and more accessible for users who rely on mobility aids such as walkers or wheelchairs. Strategic use of color contrast helps visually identify barriers, fixtures, and equipment such as the toilet, grab bars, and sinks. It aids users with vision impairments in navigating the space safely.

For **tiles**, it is recommended the use of smaller types in the shower area because it increases the amount of grout, enhancing floor grip and reducing slipping risk, particularly in wet conditions. Especially inside the shower area, installing a **built-in or retractable bench** allows users with limited endurance or mobility to sit while bathing, improving comfort and safety and eliminating the need for portable shower chairs.

Motion-activated lighting at night supports safe navigation to and from the bathroom without needing to manually switch lights on, which is particularly helpful for users with limited vision or cognition. For accessibility considerations, **drawers equipped with ergonomic, loop-style pulls** offer easier access to bathroom essentials, particularly for users with reduced hand strength or limited dexterity. In addition to the hardware, the positioning of these drawers should fall within the user's comfortable reach zone—avoiding the need to bend down excessively or stretch upward—thereby promoting both safety and independence.

Humidity sensor alerts users to excessive humidity, helping to identify areas at risk for mold and slippery conditions. It contributes to better air quality and safety by supporting preventive maintenance. Well-distributed **artificial lighting** is important for task performance and spatial awareness, especially in the shower and mirror areas. It enhances safety and comfort, particularly during hygiene routines. Although there may be regulations regarding the positioning and location of **grab bars**, it is important that these devices are placed in high-risk areas so that users can rely on them in case of potential hazards while performing activities. Therefore, it is recommended to assess the activities in their proper location, as well as the most suitable heights, which can vary from person to person.

Drains must be installed both inside and outside the shower to ensure proper water removal, preventing puddles and slips in the bathroom area and with **non-slip flooring** that is essential to increase traction and reduce fall risks, especially near entryways where wet or humid conditions are more likely. Surfaces should be even, avoiding transitions or elevation changes between wet and dry areas. A gas sensor in the bathroom is critical for detecting potential gas leaks from water heaters or other equipment, especially in poorly ventilated spaces. Early detection helps prevent serious accidents such as asphyxiation or explosions.

General recommendations for bathroom design focus on **avoiding uneven surfaces** and ensuring accessibility for all users. One important consideration is the bathroom's location within the home. While it is typically situated near the bedrooms, this is not always the case. For optimal functionality, it is crucial that the bathroom is conveniently **located close to the bedroom**, as the two spaces serve complementary purposes.

The **bathroom door should ideally open outwards**, provided there is enough external space for it to open fully. If this is not feasible, alternatives like sliding doors or doors that open inward with specialized opening mechanisms can be considered. **Lever-type handles** are recommended for doors, while furniture handles should be of the handle-type for ease of use. Another key consideration is the size of the bathroom, particularly in the context of renovations or new constructions. It is important to assess whether the room's **dimensions are sufficient for the planned activities** and necessary equipment. The layout of fixtures such as the sink, toilet, and shower should be arranged based on the tasks they are intended for. In addition to ensuring that the door opens outward, installing **locks that allow for opening from both sides** is advisable, as well as assistive technologies that enable the door to be opened more easily in an emergency. Finally, using **water-resistant materials** in the bathroom helps prevent furniture deterioration, reduces the risk of accidents, and makes maintenance easier.

The bathroom stands out as one of the most critical and high-risk environments in the home, particularly for older adults and individuals with mobility or sensory limitations. The combination of slippery surfaces, tight spaces, and the physical demands of everyday hygiene routines makes this space especially prone to accidents—most notably falls, which can lead to serious injuries or a permanent loss of independence. Therefore, careful planning, design, and implementation of safety measures are essential to promote autonomy, reduce risks, and ensure comfort and accessibility for all users. In addition to design considerations, it is crucial to consider relevant **regulations and standards** when adapting or constructing a bathroom for older adults. Each country provides specific criteria through regulations for accessibility, including minimum dimensions for circulation, grab bar placement, clear floor space around fixtures, and specifications for fixtures like toilets, sinks, and showers. These standards aim to ensure safety, comfort, and usability for individuals with varying degrees of mobility and must be consulted during planning to ensure legal compliance and functional performance. By integrating features, the bathroom can transform from a hazardous area into a safe, functional, and inclusive environment. These adaptations, when thoughtfully applied, support not only the basic activities of daily living but also contribute significantly to the overall well-being, dignity, and independence of users—particularly in aging in place and universal design contexts.

12.3 DESIGN CONSIDERATIONS

Guidelines for the Bathroom are organized into categories according to safety levels, making it easier to identify and prioritize specific design attributes, as shown in Figure 12.1.

Key Points

- **Artificial, emergency, and motion-activated lighting**: ensure well-distributed artificial lighting for task visibility. Include emergency lighting for power outages and install motion-sensor night lighting to support safe nighttime navigation and reduce the risk of falls during night-time movements.
- **Permanent ventilation**: continuous ventilation is essential to maintain air quality and control humidity in this typically moist environment. If windows are not possible, install an exhaust fan system to prevent mold growth and condensation.
- **Shower enclosure**: avoid using glass doors or fabric curtains. Prefer the construction of a masonry half-wall combined with a fixed panel, which helps contain water without creating obstacles or risks associated with breakable materials. Also, inside the shower, it is important to provide a bench to support users with limited mobility, allowing for seated bathing, increased safety, and reduced fatigue.
- **Color contrast**: help users with visual impairments identify boundaries, equipment, and pathways more easily.
- **Grab bars**: install grab bars at locations that match users' actual activity challenges (e.g., entering/exiting shower, using the toilet). Placement should be based on individual user needs, not just standard positions.
- **Non-slip flooring:** use anti-slip materials, especially in wet zones. Smaller tile sizes provide more grout lines, improving traction and reducing the risk of slips.
- **Drawer with loop-style pulls**: favor the use of drawers with loop-style pulls for easier access, particularly for users with reduced hand strength or joint issues (e.g., arthritis).
- **Gas and humidity sensors**: install gas detectors (especially when water heaters are present) and humidity sensors to prevent respiratory issues, mold, or potential accidents caused by leaks or poor air quality.

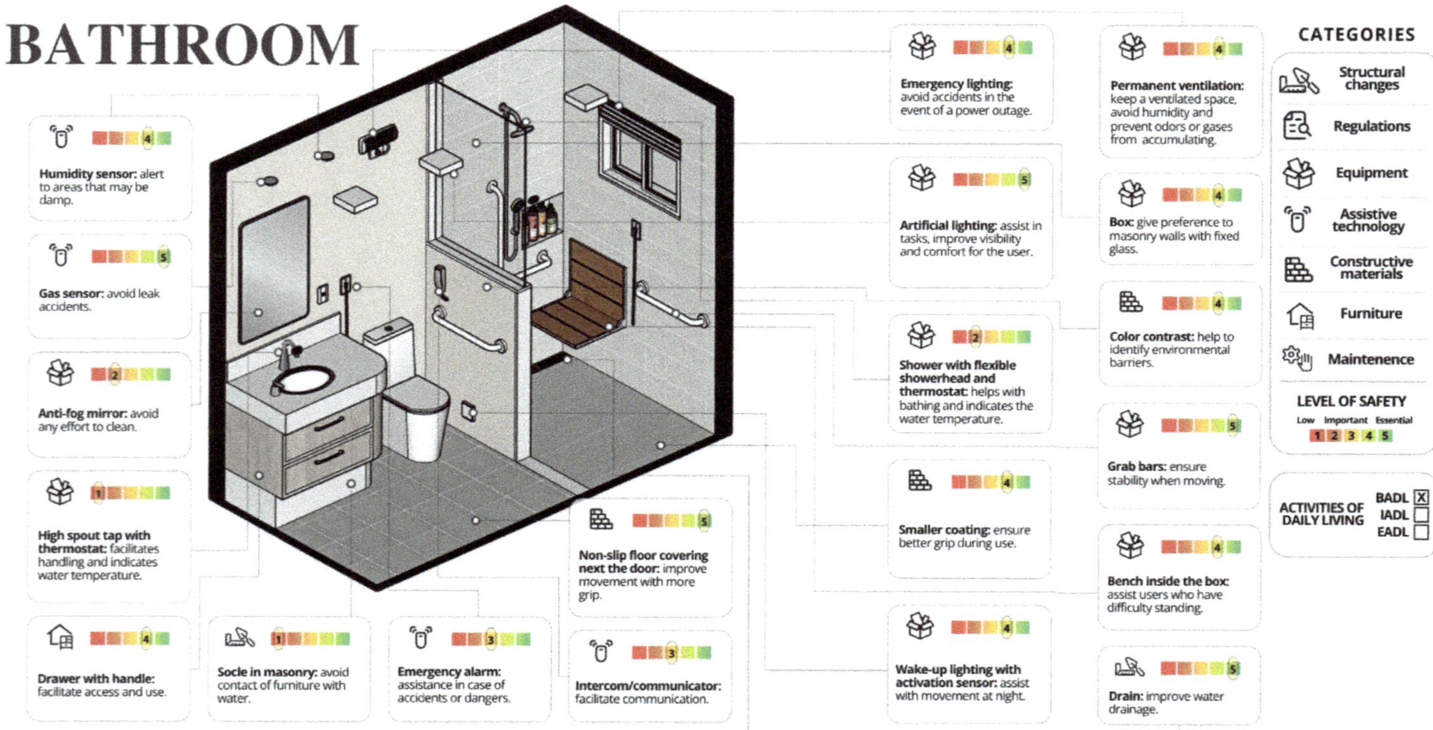

FIGURE 12.1 Design guidelines for the bathroom.

13 Bedroom

13.1 OVERVIEW OF SPACE

The bedroom serves as a space for rest, recovery, and essential daily routines. For older adults, the bedroom must be both comfortable and safe, as it is frequently used during vulnerable moments—such as waking, preparing for sleep, or moving around during the night. The physical condition in which a person wakes up can increase the risk of accidents, especially when transitioning from lying down to standing or when navigating in low-light conditions. Getting in and out of bed is a common activity that demands balance and stability, and it can pose challenges for individuals with limited mobility, reduced strength, or joint pain. Additionally, many older adults experience nighttime awakenings due to biological needs such as urinary urgency or incontinence, which often require them to walk to the bathroom. These nighttime movements can be particularly hazardous without proper lighting or support features. The types of daily activities performed in the bedroom include both basic (e.g., getting in and out of bed, dressing and undressing, sleeping or resting) and instrumental (e.g., managing medications kept on a bedside table or in drawers, using a phone or emergency alert system, preparing to safely transition to other areas of the home, such as the bathroom or living room). In addition, the bedroom often serves as a space for enhanced activities such as reading, watching television, doing crafts, and other leisure or mentally stimulating pursuits that support well-being and cognitive engagement.

13.2 SPACE COMPONENTS

The space components to improve the bathroom environment for safely aging in place are described below according to the level of safety, from minimum to maximum.

The bedroom is a private and intimate space that plays a vital role in providing individuals with a sense of security, dignity, and personal retreat. It should be designed to ensure privacy, allowing older adults to rest, dress, and carry out personal routines with comfort and autonomy. The presence of meaningful objects, photos, or decor fosters a sense of identity and emotional attachment to the space. **Personalization** supports cognitive function, comfort, and a sense of belonging—particularly important for individuals with memory loss or dementia.

Having a stable, supportive **mattress** eases the process of getting in and out of bed, especially for individuals with limited strength or balance. For **window coverings**, it is recommended that **curtains** be flame-retardant and avoid floor-length designs to reduce fire risk and prevent tripping. Simple straight models like **blinds** are recommended for ease of use and safety. Enhancing the connection between interior and exterior environments by using **windows with low sill** allows seated users to

DOI: 10.1201/9781003543701-15

view outside and contributes to psychological well-being, orientation, and a sense of inclusion in the outside world.

Matte wooden flooring reduces glare and enhances the visual perception of the floor surface, making it easier and safer to navigate, particularly for individuals with visual impairments. In the event of a fall, wood offers a warmer and softer surface compared to ceramic or tile, contributing to both physical comfort and injury prevention. Its natural texture and aesthetic also make it especially well-suited for intimate spaces like bedrooms, where a sense of warmth, quiet, and coziness is essential to well-being. **Carpeted flooring** can be a good solution, as it provides a soft and comfortable surface; however, it requires special attention due to its tendency to accumulate dust and dirt, which demands more frequent maintenance to ensure hygiene and safety.

Support bars positioned next to the bed are recommended, as they provide a secure point of leverage to assist older adults in getting up, lying down, or adjusting their position while in bed. This type of equipment can be installed between the mattress and the floor, but it is essential to ensure its stability. Therefore, when purchasing such equipment, it is important to select reliable manufacturers and verify that the products comply with current standards and regulations. Bedside support bars promote both safety and autonomy, reducing the risk of falls, minimizing the physical effort required for daily movements, and decreasing dependence on others.

Armchairs or chairs with armrests facilitate transitions between sitting and standing, providing physical support and reducing the risk of falls. Concerning assistive technologies, it is important to provide **emergency alarms** that enable immediate communication in the event of a fall, health emergency, or other dangerous situation. It ensures timely assistance while promoting a sense of independence and security. **Wake-up lighting** with an activation sensor can support nighttime movement by automatically illuminating pathways when motion is detected. It prevents disorientation or tripping when getting up during the night, especially for bathroom access.

Drawers with loop-style pulls improve accessibility to personal items, encouraging autonomy and reducing strain or frustration. The use of **contrasting colors** helps to visually differentiate surfaces, furniture, and architectural features. This is especially important for individuals with reduced vision, allowing them to better identify environmental barriers and move around with greater confidence. **Detects potential fire risks** and provides early warnings, offering critical time to respond. This is particularly important for older adults who may have slower reaction times or limited mobility.

Grab bars, when installed near the bed or along circulation routes, offer critical support for maintaining balance and stability. They are especially beneficial during transitions—such as moving from lying down to standing or navigating across the room. By providing a firm and reliable point of support, grab bars significantly reduce the risk of falls and contribute to safer, more confident mobility. For older adults, they play a key role in fostering independence, enabling them to move around the bedroom with greater security and reduced reliance on caregivers.

Adequate **lighting** improves visibility for routine activities, reduces eye strain, and enhances spatial orientation. Properly distributed lighting in the bedroom contributes significantly to both comfort and safety. In addition to other features, ensuring the safety of the bedroom environment requires specific structural adjustments. One essential recommendation is the **elimination of uneven floor levels**, which are commonly found at the transitions between rooms. These uneven surfaces can present significant barriers during both daytime and nighttime movement, increasing the risk of tripping or falls. Therefore, removing them is one of the most effective ways to promote safe and unobstructed mobility for older adults.

Accessibility to essential elements—such as the bed, light switches, furniture, and equipment—should also be carefully considered. These components must be positioned according to the user's physical abilities and limitations to encourage independence and reduce the need for assistance. Equally important is the **location of the bedroom** within the home. As an intimate and private space, it should be situated in an area that offers adequate privacy in relation to other rooms and the external environment. Additionally, solar orientation should be considered to ensure the bedroom receives comfortable levels of natural light and ventilation. This enhances thermal and environmental comfort, contributing to better rest and overall well-being.

All electrical **wiring** from equipment such as lamps, alarm clocks, and computers should be either embedded within the walls or positioned away from circulation areas to prevent tripping hazards. The bedroom **layout** should prioritize unobstructed circulation, promoting safe and independent movement. Lightweight, adaptable furniture positioned close to the walls allows users to modify the space according to their changing needs and preferences. Additionally, the bedroom should be sized appropriately to accommodate essential furniture and daily activities, ensuring both comfort and sufficient maneuverability. **Flexibility** is a key design principle in this context. Finishing materials should be **sound absorbing**, when possible, to reduce ambient noise and contribute to a peaceful atmosphere.

Accessibility to essential elements—such as the bed, light switches, furniture, and equipment—should also be carefully considered. These components must be positioned according to the user's physical abilities and limitations to encourage independence and reduce the need for assistance. All electrical **wiring** from equipment such as lamps, alarm clocks, and computers should be either embedded within the walls or positioned away from circulation areas to prevent tripping hazards.

Equally important is the **location of the bedroom** within the home. As an intimate and private space, it should be situated in an area that offers adequate privacy in relation to other rooms and the external environment. Additionally, solar orientation should be considered to ensure the bedroom receives comfortable levels of natural light and ventilation. This enhances thermal and environmental comfort, contributing to better rest and overall well-being.

One essential recommendation is the **elimination of uneven floor levels**, which are commonly found at the transitions between rooms. These uneven surfaces can present significant barriers during both daytime and nighttime movement, increasing the risk of tripping or falls. Therefore, removing them is one of the most effective ways to promote safe and unobstructed mobility for older adults.

In conclusion, the bedroom is a space at home that supports the health, safety, and independence of older adults and must be carefully planned to meet the physical, sensory, and emotional needs of its users. Given the increased vulnerability of individuals during waking hours and nighttime movements, thoughtful design is essential to reduce the risk of falls and promote confidence in independent mobility. A well-designed bedroom is not only a space of privacy and rest but also a key enabler of functional independence and quality of life.

13.3 DESIGN CONSIDERATIONS

Guidelines for the bedroom are organized into categories according to safety levels, making it easier to identify and prioritize specific design attributes, as shown in Figure 13.1.

Key Points

- **Smoke detector:** essential to provide early warning in case of fire, offering critical time for safe evacuation. This is especially important for individuals with reduced mobility or slower response times.
- **Artificial and night lighting (with motion sensor):** well-distributed artificial lighting ensures visibility for daily routines and reduces eye strain. Motion-sensor night lighting activates automatically when movement is detected, supporting safe nighttime mobility, particularly helpful during trips to the bathroom or when waking up disoriented.
- **Grab bars:** strategically placed grab bars near the bed and along circulation paths assist with balance and stability. It is useful for transitions like getting in and out of bed, reducing fall risk, and promoting independence.
- **Drawer with loop-style pulls:** drawers should feature ergonomic loop-style pulls for easier grip and use, especially by individuals with limited hand strength or dexterity. They allow safer and more comfortable access to personal items.
- **Color contrast:** applying contrasting colors to walls, furniture, and floors helps visually differentiate surfaces and elements. This is important for users with vision impairments, enabling safer navigation and reducing confusion or disorientation.

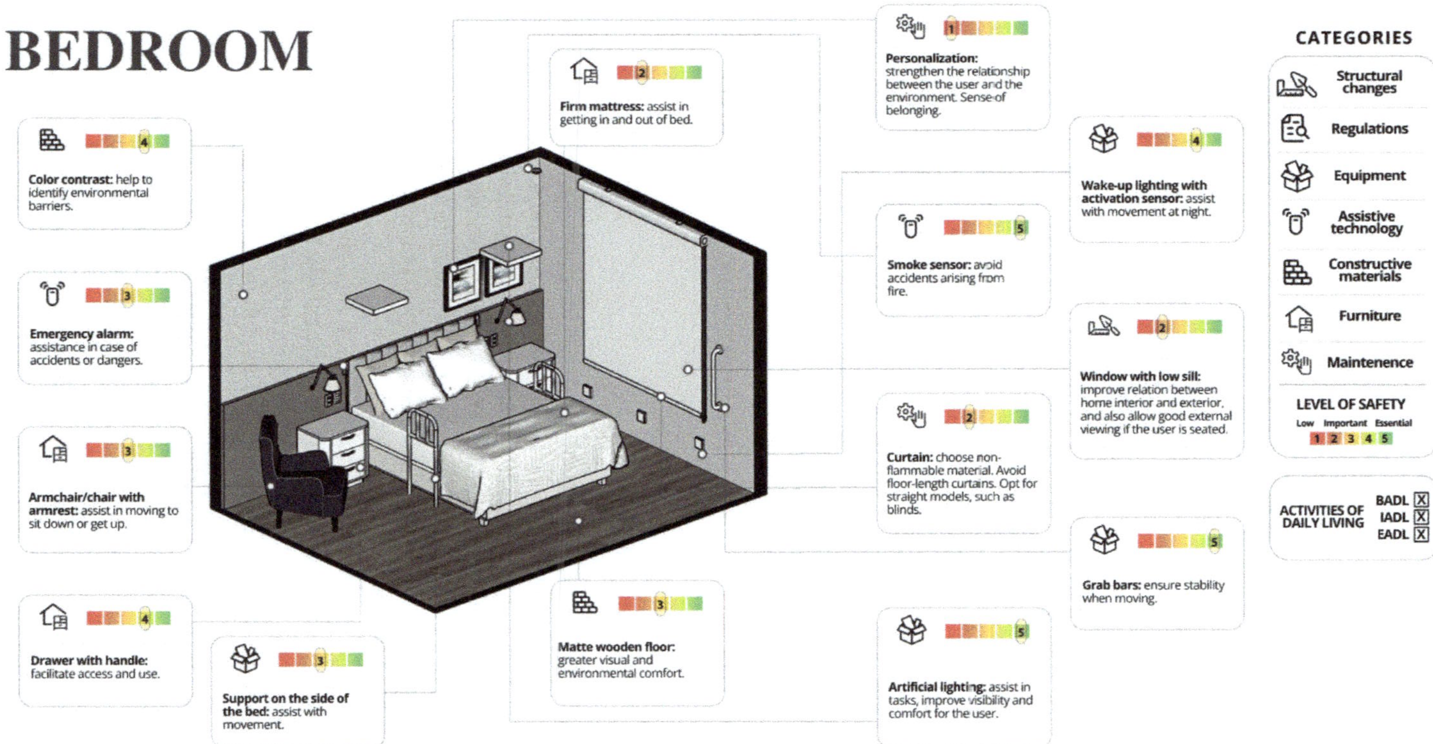

FIGURE 13.1 Design guidelines for the bedroom.

14 Closet

14.1 OVERVIEW OF SPACE

The closet is a practical yet meaningful space in the home, primarily designed for storing clothing and personal items. For older adults, it plays a vital role in maintaining independence and supporting daily self-care routines. This space is typically where basic activities of daily living (BADLs) are performed (e.g., getting dressed or undressed, and selecting appropriate attire based on weather, activity, or time of day). These seemingly simple tasks can become increasingly challenging with age due to mobility limitations, decreased flexibility, or cognitive decline, making the design and organization of the closet especially important. Beyond its functional role, the closet can also support enhanced activities of daily living (EADLs), including interactions with caregivers or family members who are involved such as assisting an older adult in selecting an outfit for a special occasion or helping organize seasonal clothing provides opportunities for meaningful social connection. These shared moments not only support daily functioning but also foster a sense of dignity, autonomy, and engagement—key components of aging in place with quality of life. Designing the closet with accessibility in mind can greatly enhance its usability and transform it into a supportive, personalized environment that meets the evolving needs of older adults.

14.2 SPACE COMPONENTS

The space components to improve the closet environment for safely aging in place are described below according to the level of safety, from minimum to maximum.

To ensure a minimum level of safety elements such as **curtains,** when used, must be made of non-flammable material to reduce fire risks, avoiding floor-length designs for safety. When specifying tall cabinets, it is essential to incorporate **pull-down closet rods** to enhance accessibility, allowing users to reach and operate them effortlessly and without strain.

Mirrors should be integrated into the design thoughtfully, as they can significantly enhance spatial perception, which is especially beneficial for older adults. Strategically placing mirrors at varying heights allows individuals to better gauge their surroundings and navigate their environment more confidently. Mirrors play a practical role in daily activities, such as dressing, grooming, or helping users see areas that may otherwise be difficult to reach or monitor. For example, large full-length mirrors can provide a broader view of the individual's appearance, while smaller well-positioned mirrors can aid in tasks like putting on shoes or adjusting clothing. Beyond functionality, mirrors contribute to creating a sense of openness and light within the space, making the closet feel larger and more accessible.

DOI: 10.1201/9781003543701-16

By incorporating **supportive benches** within the closet space can provide significant benefits for individuals with mobility challenges. These benches offer a stable and comfortable seating option, allowing users to take a rest while dressing, putting on shoes, or simply organizing their clothing. For those with limited mobility, such as individuals who use walkers or wheelchairs, a bench serves as a practical support that aids in balance and helps reduce the strain of prolonged standing. It allows users to sit while adjusting, improving overall comfort and independence in daily activities. Ideally, the bench should be at a height that accommodates a variety of users and can be integrated with additional storage options, such as drawers or shelves beneath it, to further maximize space efficiency.

Windows with low sills are a valuable feature that improves both the functionality and the aesthetic of the space. A low sill allows seated individuals—whether they are sitting on a bench or in a wheelchair—to have an unobstructed view of the outdoors without the need to stand or strain. Additionally, a low sill ensures that natural light can enter the space more easily, enhancing visibility and making the closet feel brighter and more inviting. This small design choice contributes to greater independence and ease of use, especially for those who may have difficulty standing for extended periods. However, privacy is also an important consideration in such spaces. To maintain a balance between access to natural light and privacy, it is recommended to use curtains, as previously discussed.

Built-in lighting within closets plays a crucial role in enhancing ambient lighting, significantly improving visibility and making it easier to locate and organize items. The choice of flooring is equally important for both comfort and safety. **Artificial lighting** should be integrated throughout the closet to support daily tasks, ensuring that users can clearly see and reach the items they need without difficulty. Bright, even lighting not only aids in functionality but also creates a welcoming and well-organized environment. **Wake-up lighting** equipped with a motion sensor is an essential feature for nighttime movement, automatically illuminating the space when it detects movement. This ensures that users can move safely and comfortably without fumbling for switches, particularly during the night when visibility is limited.

A **matte wooden floor** is highly recommended as it offers both visual and environmental comfort. The matte finish reduces glare, which can be disorienting, particularly in bright light conditions, and minimizes reflections that might interfere with the user's ability to see clearly. Additionally, the textured surface of matte wood provides enhanced traction, which is crucial for preventing slips and falls, especially for individuals with mobility challenges or those prone to balance issues. The natural warmth and aesthetic appeal of wood also contribute to a calming, inviting atmosphere within the space.

An **emergency alarm** system should be integrated into the design to ensure a quick response in case of accidents. The alarm should be easily accessible and loud enough to alert individuals nearby, providing peace of mind to both the user and caregivers. To further enhance safety, it is highly recommended to include **emergency lighting** in the closet. This lighting will automatically activate during power outages, ensuring that the user has adequate illumination to navigate the space and avoid accidents. The emergency lights should be strategically placed to ensure they provide adequate coverage across the entire closet area, highlighting potential hazards and obstacles.

Incorporating **color contrast** into the design can also greatly improve navigation. By using contrasting colors on the edges of shelves, drawers, and cabinet handles, users can better distinguish between different elements within the closet. For example, contrasting colors on the floor or shelving can draw attention to the boundaries of the space, helping individuals with limited vision or those unfamiliar with the layout navigate with greater ease and confidence. This simple yet effective design strategy can highlight potential environmental barriers, such as uneven floors or corners, making the space safer and more intuitive to use.

Drawers with loop-style pulls are another practical addition, designed to improve ease of access to stored items. It eliminates the need for complicated or strenuous maneuvers, allowing users to open and close drawers with minimal effort, which is especially important for individuals with limited hand strength or mobility challenges.

A **smoke detector** is a safety feature, providing early warning of potential fire hazards that might otherwise go unnoticed. This gives older adults the ability to respond quickly in case of an emergency, improving their safety and peace of mind. Finally, **grab bars** should be strategically placed within the closet space to provide support and stability while moving around. These bars help prevent falls and enhance confidence, making it easier for users to navigate the area with greater security.

Other recommendations for this space also relate to its overall **planning and layout**. It is essential to design a furniture and equipment arrangement that promotes safe, autonomous, and comfortable use of the area. **Circulation zones should be free** of physical barriers, ensuring easy and hazard-free movement. When selecting furniture, it's important to choose pieces with **rounded edges**, as sharp corners can pose a risk of injury. Additionally, handles and drawer slides should be specified to allow for easy operation, particularly for individuals with reduced strength or dexterity. It is also advisable to **avoid the use of loose rugs** and **exposed electrical cords**, as these can create tripping hazards and compromise safety.

Designing a closet that is functional, accessible, and safe is essential for supporting older adults in maintaining their independence and dignity as they age in place. Thoughtfully integrating safety features ensures that this space not only supports daily routines like dressing but helps to minimize physical strain and the risk of accidents. Additionally, attention to details such as seating, color contrast, and visual access to the outside contributes to both physical and emotional well-being. When combined with appropriate layout planning and barrier-free circulation, the closet transforms from a simple storage area into a supportive, empowering space that respects the needs and capabilities of its users.

14.3 DESIGN CONSIDERATIONS

Guidelines for the closet are organized into categories according to safety levels, making it easier to identify and prioritize specific design attributes, as shown in Figure 14.1.

Key Points

- **Artificial lighting:** should be well distributed to ensure proper visibility for all closet-related tasks. Install motion-activated night lighting is also essential for detecting presence during nighttime, providing safety without the need to use switches and emergency lighting to ensure visibility during power outages, reducing the risk of accidents.
- **Grab bars:** although not commonly used in closets, should be strategically placed to help maintain balance while dressing or putting on shoes, enhancing safety.
- **Smoke detectors:** essential to quickly identify fire hazards, enabling immediate response and improving safety.
- **Drawers with loop-style pulls:** make it easier for individuals with reduced strength or dexterity to operate, improving accessibility.
- **Color contrast:** should be used between floors, handles, drawers, and shelves to improve element recognition and navigation, especially for people with low vision.

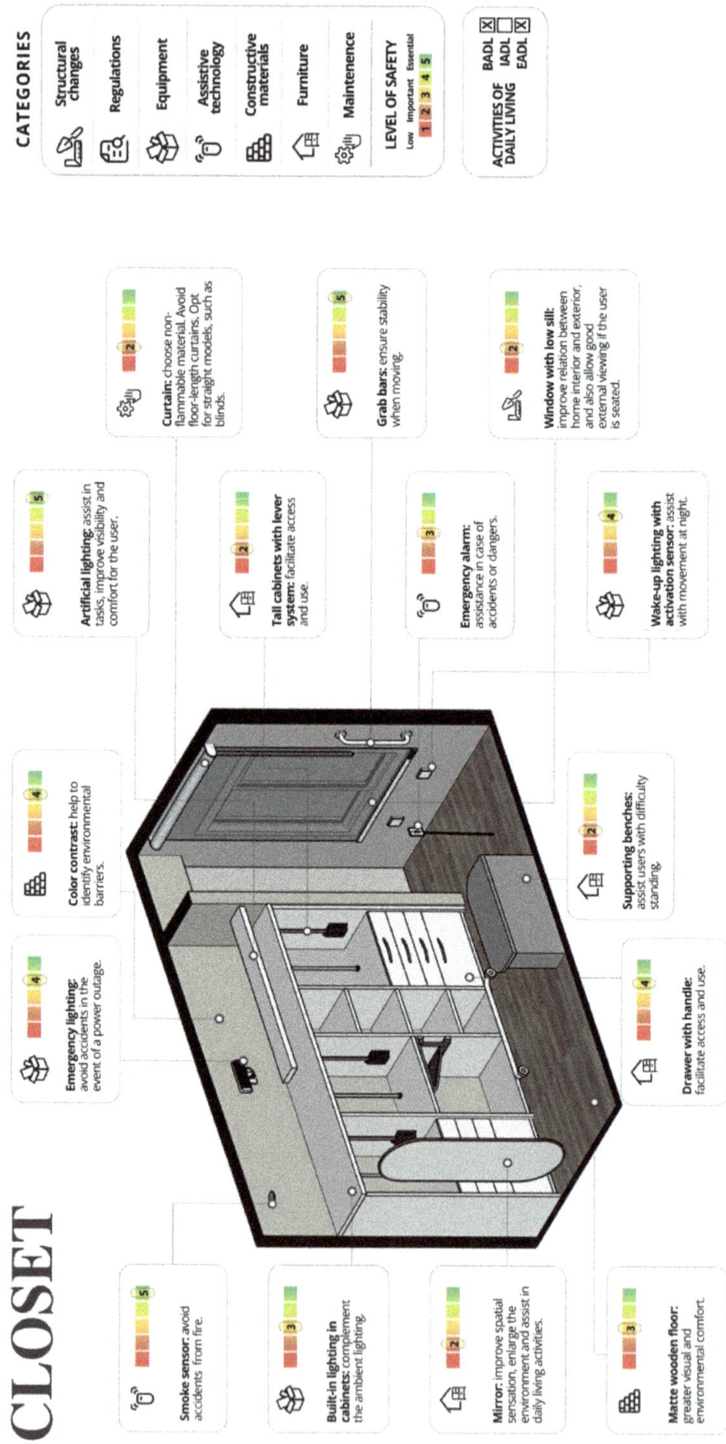

FIGURE 14.1 Design guidelines for the closet.

15 Home Office

15.1 OVERVIEW OF SPACE

The profile of older adults has changed considerably in recent decades. Unlike previous generations, today's older adults are typically more active, independent, and engaged in a wide range of social, intellectual, and even professional activities. Many continue to work part-time, volunteer, or pursue personal projects well into retirement. This evolution reflects a growing emphasis on maintaining autonomy, purpose, and a high quality of life throughout the aging process. As a result, there is an increasing need for environments that are not only safe but also thoughtfully designed to support this dynamic lifestyle. A well-adapted living space plays a crucial role in enabling older adults to carry out their daily routines with confidence, comfort, and minimal risk. Such spaces should address both the physical and cognitive demands of aging while reinforcing a sense of dignity and self-sufficiency. In this context, older adults typically perform at their home office instrumental (e.g., handling finances, doing housework, shopping, and using communication devices) and enhanced (engaging in hobbies, using technology for communication or entertainment, attending social gatherings, and participating in lifelong learning) activities of daily living. Supporting these activities contributes to emotional well-being, mental stimulation, and social inclusion.

15.2 SPACE COMPONENTS

The space components of the home office are organized in this chapter from the minimum to maximum level of safety.

Creating a sense of **personalization** is essential. Incorporating familiar objects, family photos, meaningful decorations, or cherished mementos helps reinforce the individual's emotional connection to the space. This personalization transforms a functional work area into a comforting environment, fostering a sense of identity, belonging, and psychological well-being. It can also enhance focus and motivation by making the space feel welcoming and personally relevant. Special attention for window treatments like **curtains and blinds** that must be chosen not only for aesthetic appeal but also for safety and practicality. It is highly recommended to use non-flammable materials to reduce fire risk as well as to avoid floor-length curtains, which may become tripping hazards—especially if mobility aids are in use. Opting for streamlined, easy-to-operate options such as vertical or roller blinds ensures greater ease of use and minimizes clutter, supporting a safer and more accessible work environment. **Windows with low sills** are particularly beneficial in a home office. They not only allow more natural light into the home but also enable seated individuals to enjoy external views. This fosters a connection with the outdoors, which can be mentally stimulating and emotionally uplifting.

DOI: 10.1201/9781003543701-17

Armchairs or chairs with armrests are important for promoting mobility and physical autonomy for older adults. These features offer stable support during the transitional movements of sitting down and standing up—actions that can become increasingly difficult with age due to reduced muscle strength, joint stiffness, or balance issues. The presence of armrests allows individuals to distribute their weight more evenly and use their upper body to assist with movement, significantly reducing the strain placed on the knees, hips, and lower back. When selecting such seating for a home office, it is important to consider factors like appropriate seat height, firmness of the cushion, and sturdy armrest construction, all of which further enhance comfort and usability.

An emergency alarm system allows the user to call for help in the event of an accident or health emergency. This technology brings peace of mind to both the elderly person and their family, ensuring help is always within reach. When it comes to flooring, **matte wooden surfaces** are recommended because they reduce glare and are generally less slippery than glossy finishes. Additionally, they enhance visual and environmental comfort. The **use of carpets or loose rugs are discouraged** as they can become tripping hazards, especially when mobility aids such as canes or walkers are used.

For ease of use, **drawers with loop-style pulls** are preferred. They require less effort to open and close, making them ideal for older adults who may experience reduced grip strength or arthritis. **Tables and chairs with straight legs** help minimize the risk of tripping. Furniture with complex or angled legs can become hazards, especially when using mobility aids such as canes or walkers. One essential feature is the use of **color contrast**, which significantly aids in identifying environmental barriers. High contrast between walls, floors, and furniture improves visual clarity, helping elderly individuals navigate their homes more safely—particularly important for those experiencing visual decline.

Emergency lighting is an important consideration. In the event of a power outage, these lights provide immediate illumination, helping elderly residents avoid disorientation and potential falls. The installation of a **smoke sensor** is a crucial safety measure. These devices can detect the early signs of fire, giving residents the opportunity to respond quickly. For elderly individuals who may have limited mobility or slower reaction times, this can be lifesaving.

Installing **grab bars** in strategic locations, such as bathrooms and hallways, provides stability and support. These are essential for preventing falls and offering physical reassurance during movement, especially when navigating. Proper **artificial lighting** is essential in a home office, particularly for older adults who may experience age-related changes in vision, such as reduced contrast sensitivity or increased sensitivity to glare. Well-designed, strategically placed lighting enhances visibility, reduces eye strain during prolonged reading or computer use, and contributes to a more comfortable and productive workspace. In a home office environment, task lighting such as adjustable desk lamps should be used to illuminate specific areas where close-up work is performed. Ambient lighting should be evenly distributed to avoid harsh shadows, while indirect light sources can soften the atmosphere and reduce glare on screens. It is also beneficial to choose lighting with adjustable brightness and color temperature to accommodate different times of day and personal preferences. Beyond improving visual comfort, proper lighting also plays a role in safety. Even within the office, poor lighting can increase the risk of tripping over cords, furniture, or uneven flooring. Ensuring clear, consistent illumination throughout the space helps prevent accidents and supports confident movement.

The positioning and location of the home office within the house should also be carefully considered. Just like a bedroom, this space benefits from being placed in a quiet, private area, away from the main circulation zones of the home. Minimizing noise and external interruptions supports focus and concentration, which are essential for productive work or administrative tasks.

Furniture layout is another critical aspect of home office safety and functionality. All pieces should be arranged to allow for unobstructed circulation, especially for individuals with reduced mobility. Considering flexibility supports both ergonomic adjustments and evolving user needs. Acoustic comfort should also be considered. The use of **materials with sound-absorbing** properties, such as acoustic panels, curtains, or wall coverings, can significantly reduce echo and noise disturbance. Finally, it is important to align the **size of the room with its intended function.** An office that is too cramped can limit movement and increase the risk of accidents, while an excessively large space may require additional lighting and heating, reducing efficiency. A well-proportioned room ensures not only a higher level of safety but also encourages regular use by providing a comfortable, functional, and adaptable work environment.

The design for a home office for older adults requires a thoughtful balance between functionality, comfort, and safety due to the fact that today, older adults lead increasingly active and engaged lives, and their home environments must adapt to support both their physical needs and their evolving roles in society. A well-designed workspace not only enhances productivity but also fosters independence, autonomy, emotional well-being, and cognitive stimulation. By minimizing physical barriers, supporting sensory and mobility limitations, and reinforcing a sense of identity and purpose, the home office becomes more than a place to complete tasks. As part of a broader strategy for aging in place, such environments play a crucial role in promoting quality of life and enabling older adults to remain active, connected, and fulfilled in their daily lives.

15.3 DESIGN CONSIDERATIONS

Guidelines for the home office are organized into categories according to safety levels, making it easier to identify and prioritize specific design attributes, as shown in Figure 15.1.

Key Points

- **Drawers with loop-style pulls:** prefer drawers with loop-style pulls, which are easier to grip and ideal for individuals with arthritis or reduced hand strength.
- **Grab bars:** install grab bars in strategic locations such as near seating areas and along circulation paths to provide support, improve balance, and reduce the risk of falls.

- **Tables and chairs with straight legs:** choose furniture with straight, stable legs to reduce tripping hazards. Avoid angled or decorative legs that may obstruct mobility aids. It is important to avoid swivel or wheeled chairs. Rolling chairs can be unstable and increase fall risk. Opt for fixed chairs with armrests to support safe sitting and standing.
- **General artificial and emergency lighting:** ensure well-distributed ambient lighting to reduce shadows and improve visibility. Install emergency lighting to activate during power outages for safe navigation.
- **Color contrast:** use contrasting colors between floors, walls, and furniture to aid visual perception and help individuals with low vision distinguish objects and surfaces more easily.
- **Smoke detector:** install smoke sensors to detect fire hazards early and provide enough time for evacuation, which is especially crucial for users with limited mobility or slower reaction times.

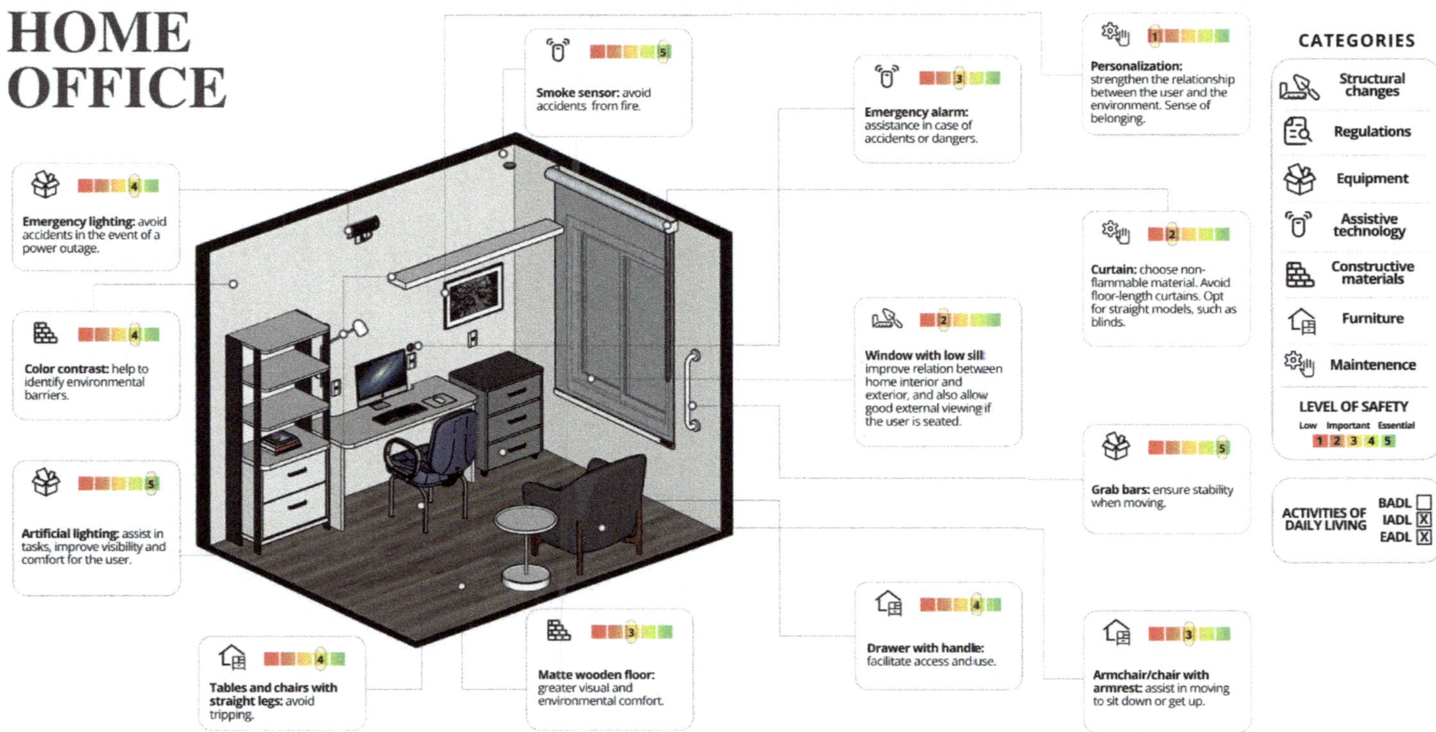

FIGURE 15.1 Design guidelines for the home office.

16 Other Spaces

16.1 OVERVIEW

The earlier chapters focused on the spaces that are found in many homes or apartments. In this chapter we discuss several other spaces that would benefit from design guidance to improve safety for older adults. These other spaces include the garage, exercise room, and outdoor areas, all of which play a vital role in supporting safety, mobility, and overall well-being for older adults aging in place.

The recommendations of these spaces are more general in nature and do not adhere to the same level of safety detail provided for other environments discussed earlier in this book. It is important to emphasize that the design of these areas, as well as any potential environmental modifications, should consider the users' specific needs related to how they use the space, along with their abilities and limitations in performing daily tasks. In this section, we present a series of recommendations designed to enhance the safety of these areas in activities of daily living.

16.2 GARAGE

When designing or adapting a garage for use by older adults, it is essential to incorporate space components to support mobility, independence, and accident prevention. One of the primary concerns is the **avoidance of floor level changes**. Even if the garage is an open or semi-covered structure, the floor should be gently sloped toward drains to facilitate water runoff. In cases of significant level changes, it is advisable to install **ramps** designed in accordance with each country's regulations on dimensions and inclination.

The installation of **smoke and gas detectors** is crucial, especially in enclosed garages where the accumulation of fumes or undetected gas leaks can pose serious health risks. These detectors should be positioned according to safety guidelines and regularly maintained to ensure proper functioning. Adequate **artificial lighting** must be provided to ensure visibility at all times of day. This includes **emergency lighting**, which is essential during power outages. Light switches and electrical outlets should be positioned at accessible heights to accommodate users of varying physical abilities.

The use of **non-slip flooring** materials is strongly recommended to reduce the risk of falls, particularly when the floor is wet. Additionally, incorporating **contrast colors** between the floor, walls, and structural elements (like steps or ramps) helps visually impaired users navigate the space more safely.

Handrails or support bars should be installed along pathways, near steps, and in areas where additional support might be required when entering or exiting vehicles. These assistive elements help guide safe movement and provide physical stability. **Installing motion-sensor lighting** is another valuable strategy, particularly for older

DOI: 10.1201/9781003543701-18

adults who may enter the garage with hands full or have limited dexterity. This feature not only adds convenience but also increases the level of safety by automatically illuminating the space as someone approaches.

In an enclosed garage, exhaust fans should be used to maintain air quality. These systems help eliminate harmful gases and unpleasant odors, contributing to a healthier indoor environment. Additional safety features can be incorporated into the garage environment. These may include an **emergency alarm system** that allows the user to call for assistance in case of an accident or health issue. **Automated door systems** that enable remote or hands-free opening and closing of the garage door improve accessibility and convenience for individuals with reduced mobility. **Water-resistant and low-maintenance surface materials for floors and walls** not only enhance durability but also facilitate easy cleaning and hygiene maintenance. In garage areas, it is equally important to incorporate properly **placed drainage systems** to ensure efficient water runoff, prevent puddling, and maintain a dry, safe surface—especially in spaces exposed to vehicle washing, rainwater, or accidental spills. By addressing these design elements, the garage can become a safe, functional, and accessible space that accommodates the specific needs of older adults, whether they are drivers, passengers, or simply passing through the area. Thoughtful planning ensures the environment supports both daily routines and emergency situations, promoting overall well-being and autonomy.

Key Points

- **Avoidance of floor level changes:** prevents tripping hazards and supports safe, easy movement for older adults, especially those using wheelchairs or walkers. A smooth, continuous surface ensures better accessibility and safer transfers in and out of vehicles.
- **Non-slip flooring**: install anti-slip surfaces to reduce the risk of falls, especially in areas exposed to water or low lighting.
- **Artificial lighting:** include both artificial and emergency lighting to improve visibility and safety, especially at night or during power outages. Use presence sensors for automatic activation.
- **Smoke and gas detectors:** it is important to alert older adults to fires or gas leaks, preventing serious health risks and ensuring a safer environment.
- **Emergency alarm system:** allows older adults to quickly call for help in case of an accident or health issue.

16.3 EXERCISE ROOM

Physical exercise is very important for older adults to maintain health and prevent accidents. Regular activity helps improve strength, flexibility, balance, and coordination, all of which are essential for daily functioning. Therefore, creating a safe and supportive exercise environment encourages consistent use and promotes overall well-being. Whenever possible, physical activities should be supervised by a qualified professional to ensure safety, proper technique, and to provide assistance if needed.

When designing or adapting an exercise room for use by older adults, it is essential to incorporate space components that support mobility, independence, and accident prevention. One of the primary concerns is ensuring **adequate space** for safe movement and exercise equipment use. There should be clear, **unobstructed pathways** around all equipment to allow wheelchair or walker access and to reduce the risk of tripping or falling. The **flooring** in an exercise room should be firm, even, and **slip-resistant** to provide stability during physical activity. Shock-absorbing materials, such as cushioned vinyl or rubber flooring, can reduce joint strain and the impact of accidental falls. It is important to ensure a level, even floor surface to prevent trips and falls.

Artificial lighting is crucial to ensure visibility and safety at all times. Light switches should be installed at accessible heights, and motion-sensor lighting can be considered for ease of use. Mirrors can be strategically placed to support proper exercise form and alignment, but they should not create confusing reflections or glare. **Continuous ventilation** is another important consideration to maintain comfortable temperatures and good air quality, especially during physical exertion.

Handrails or support bars along walls or near exercise equipment can provide additional stability and confidence, especially during balance or flexibility exercises. **Contrast colors** between the floor, walls, and exercise equipment can improve navigation and reduce visual confusion, particularly for users with low vision. Storage solutions should be designed to keep the space organized and free from clutter, with shelves and racks positioned at accessible heights. An **emergency alarm system** or call button should be installed within easy reach to allow users to request assistance in case of an accident or health issue. **Water-resistant and easy-to-clean materials** for floors and equipment surfaces facilitate hygiene maintenance, which is especially important in shared environments. All materials and equipment should be positioned within each **user's reach envelope** and tailored to their individual needs and limitations.

By addressing these design elements, the exercise room can become a safe, functional, and inviting space that accommodates the specific needs of older adults. Thoughtful planning ensures that the environment not only supports physical activity to maintain strength, flexibility, balance, and coordination but also promotes health, reduces the risk of falls, and enhances independence and quality of life.

Key Points

- **Non-slip flooring with shock-absorbing materials:** essential to prevent slips and falls during physical activity. It provides stable footing, especially when users may sweat or if the floor becomes damp, reducing the risk of injuries.
- **Handrails or support bars:** provide essential stability, supporting safer movement and greater confidence during exercise for older adults.
- **Unobstructed pathway:** ensure safe and easy movement around equipment, especially for older adults using wheelchairs, walkers, or other mobility aids.
- **Emergency alarm system**: allows older adults to quickly call for help if they experience an accident, fall, or health issue.

- **Artificial lighting:** include both artificial and emergency lighting to improve visibility and safety, especially at night or during power outages. Use presence sensors for automatic activation.
- **Color contrast:** helps in identifying environmental barriers

16.4 OUTDOOR AREAS

Outdoor areas—such as gardens, poolside areas, and social gathering spaces—can significantly enhance the quality of life for older adults when thoughtfully designed with accessibility, safety, and comfort in mind. These spaces, when properly planned, not only offer opportunities for relaxation and social interaction but also support autonomy, mobility, and overall well-being.

To ensure safety and usability, several essential features should be incorporated. Circulation paths must be equipped with sturdy **handrails or support bars**, particularly in areas with inclines, curves, or level transitions. These provide crucial support and stability, especially for individuals who use walking aids or experience balance difficulties. **Outdoor flooring should be finished with non-slip materials**, ideally using small-tile flooring to maximize grout lines and enhance traction. In areas prone to moisture, such as around pools or garden irrigation systems, these materials help to reduce the risk of slips and falls even in wet conditions.

Lighting plays an important role in creating a secure outdoor environment. **Motion-sensor lights** that activate upon detecting movement can enhance nighttime safety while eliminating the need to locate switches in the dark. Additionally, **emergency lighting** should be installed to ensure visibility during power outages. **Proper drainage** systems are also critical—outdoor surfaces should be subtly graded to direct water toward well-placed drains, minimizing the formation of puddles that could pose slipping hazards.

Functional features that promote ease and peace of mind should be considered. For instance, an **intercom** system between outdoor and indoor areas allows for quick and easy communication, reducing the need for potentially exhausting or unsafe trips back inside. Strategically placed rest areas with water-resistant **benches or seating**—featuring straight legs, and rounded edges and armrests—offer comfortable spots for breaks and support safe transitions between sitting and standing. Furthermore, clearly accessible **emergency alarm systems** should be installed throughout outdoor zones to provide immediate assistance in the event of a fall, health emergency, or other danger.

Equally important is the avoidance of common design hazards such as **steps and abrupt changes** in elevation and, when necessary, replaced with gentle **ramps** that include **handrails** and **textured surfaces to enhance grip and stability**. This recommendation is especially relevant in outdoor areas, where ramps should be prioritized over steps or level differences—even minimal ones—whenever possible. Ramps allow for smoother and safer transitions and are generally more suitable for individuals with mobility challenges. In these cases, it is essential to consult the applicable **regulations and standards in each country regarding ramp inclination and dimensions** to ensure compliance and user safety.

Loose or **exposed electrical cables**—used for lighting, irrigation, or sound systems—**must be securely concealed to prevent tripping risks** and maintain a clean, navigable space. By integrating these strategies, outdoor areas in homes for older adults can become not only safe and accessible but also welcoming, inclusive, and enriching. A well-designed outdoor environment supports freedom of movement, encourages engagement with nature, and fosters opportunities for meaningful social connection—all of which are essential elements in promoting both physical and emotional health in later life.

Key Points

- **Non-slip flooring**: crucial to prevent slips and falls, especially when surfaces are wet from rain, dew, or cleaning. Preference for small-tile flooring. Non-slip flooring provides better traction for older adults, enhancing safety and confidence when walking or using mobility aids outdoors.
- **Accessibility-compliant ramp**: incorporate ramps designed according to each country's accessibility regulations and principles of universal design, ensuring safe and easy access for all users.
- **Handrails or support bars**: provide stability and prevent falls, helping older adults move safely and confidently.
- **Artificial lighting**: include both artificial and emergency lighting to improve visibility and safety, especially at night or during power outages. Use presence sensors for automatic activation.

16.5 CONCLUSIONS

This chapter highlights the importance of considering additional spaces in the home environment, which may be common in some living environments but not found in all. Moreover, there may be spaces that we have not discussed here that are used by older adults, such as a dedicated craft room, a carport, a game room, or a library. Importantly, the strategies discussed here should be adapted to the specific needs, abilities, and preferences of each individual, ensuring that all environmental modifications are meaningful and supportive of their daily routines and activities. The approach we have taken in this chapter, and throughout the book, provides a guide for the processes that should be followed when evaluating spaces where older adults spend their time. The categories provide a framework for review of the components of each space and the topics for assessment of safety. Ultimately, the aim is to create environments that not only meet basic needs but also enrich daily life, encourage active engagement, and empower older adults to live with dignity, comfort, and confidence in their own homes.

Section III

Final Considerations

17 General Guidelines

The complete set of guidelines from the book are presented in **Table 17.1**, organized by categories for each housing environment. This summary consolidates all space components discussed throughout Chapters 7 to 16, offering a comprehensive overview of the recommendations previously outlined. By presenting the information in a clear and structured format, the table enables stakeholders to quickly identify how each directive applies to specific environments and categories.

This synthesized format not only promotes consistency in design and decision-making but also serves as a valuable foundation for the development of checklists aimed at evaluating and improving residential spaces. Although the focus of this work is on enhancing safety and usability for older adults, many of the proposed modifications contribute to broader usability and accessibility, benefiting people of all ages and abilities. As such, the guidelines support the creation of inclusive and universally safer home environments.

In the first column are the **categories for home improvement**, and the second column outlines the corresponding **space components**. Columns three through eleven represent the various **housing spaces**, allowing for a cross-referenced view of how each recommendation applies across different areas of the home.

TABLE 17.1
Summary of Space Components for Safe Housing Environment

		Categories											
Categories	**Guidelines**	**Front door**	**Living room**	**Dining room**	**Kitchen**	**Laundry room**	**Bathroom**	**Bedroom**	**Closet**	**Home office**	**Garage**	**Exercise room**	**Outdoor areas**
Structural changes	Ramps: facilitate the transition between different floor levels. Meet legal requirements	♦									♦		♦
	Entrance hall: provides privacy between the entryway and the rest of the home	♦											
	Room location: avoid placing noisy environments near areas that require greater sound privacy		♦	♦	♦	♦	♦	♦	♦	♦			
	Drain: ensures proper water drainage	♦				♦	♦				♦		♦
	Uneven surfaces: differences between wet and dry areas should be managed using flooring patterns that indicate slopes toward drains	♦				♦	♦				♦		♦

(Continued)

DOI: 10.1201/9781003543701-20

TABLE 17.1 *(Continued)*
Summary of Space Components for Safe Housing Environment

Categories	Guidelines	Front door	Living room	Dining room	Kitchen	Laundry room	Bathroom	Bedroom	Closet	Home office	Garage	Exercise room	Outdoor areas
Structural changes	Electrical outlet protection: prevents accidents when outlets are used after exposure to moisture						♦						
	Embedded rugs in the floor: prevent tripping hazards	♦											
	Low sill windows: improve the connection between indoor and outdoor spaces	♦	♦	♦				♦	♦	♦			
	Socle in masonry: protects furniture from water damage, improves hygiene. It is durable, easy to clean, and prevents dampness				♦	♦	♦						
Regulations	Dimensional regulations: ensure minimum dimensions for functional spaces and circulation areas in accordance with applicable standards	♦	♦	♦	♦	♦	♦	♦	♦	♦	♦	♦	♦
Equipment	Support bars/handrails: assist users in moving through circulation areas and indoor spaces, providing support and stability	♦	♦	♦	♦	♦	♦	♦	♦	♦	♦	♦	♦
	Accessibility adjustments: switches, furniture, appliances, and objects should be positioned within each user's reach envelope, accounting for their abilities and potential motor limitations	♦	♦	♦	♦	♦	♦	♦	♦	♦			
	Artificial lighting (general or task-specific): should be positioned to assist in task execution, providing benefits such as improved visibility and user comfort	♦	♦	♦	♦	♦	♦	♦	♦	♦	♦	♦	♦
	Emergency lighting: prevents accidents during power outages	♦	♦	♦	♦	♦	♦		♦	♦	♦	♦	♦
	Anti-fog mirrors: eliminate the need for users to wipe mirrors manually						♦						
	Loop-style pulls: facilitate grip		♦	♦	♦	♦	♦	♦	♦	♦			

TABLE 17.1 *(Continued)*
Summary of Space Components for Safe Housing Environment

Categories	Guidelines	Front door	Living room	Dining room	Kitchen	Laundry room	Bathroom	Bedroom	Closet	Home office	Garage	Exercise room	Outdoor areas
	Built-in cabinet lighting: complements general artificial lighting		♦		♦				♦				
	Continuous ventilation or exhaust fan: air circulation and renewal, as well as natural lighting. When this is not possible, install an exhaust fan				♦	♦	♦				♦	♦	
	Sound-absorbing materials: minimize noise and echo, enhancing acoustics and creating a more peaceful, comfortable environment		♦	♦				♦		♦			
	Lever-type door handles: facilitate ease of use and grip for users on doors that provide access to different spaces	♦	♦	♦	♦	♦	♦	♦	♦	♦			
	Emergency contact information: should be placed in a visible location in case of accidents				♦								
	Personalization: strengthens place attachment		♦	♦				♦		♦			
	Support benches: assist individuals who have difficulty standing for extended periods								♦				
Equipment	Heated towel racks: facilitate towel drying						♦						
	Induction cooktop: reduces the risk of burns and eliminates gas handling				♦								
	Retractable drying rack: should be placed in a way that does not obstruct movement					♦							
	Dual-sided door lock: allows the door to be opened from both inside and outside for accessibility and safety						♦						
	Flexible shower head with a thermostat: allow precise temperature control and easy adjustment, making bathing more accessible						♦						
	Water thermostat: visually indicates temperature				♦	♦	♦						
	Support bar on the side of the bed: assist the individuals getting in and out of bed, while preventing falls during sleep							♦					

(Continued)

TABLE 17.1 *(Continued)*
Summary of Space Components for Safe Housing Environment

Categories	Guidelines	Front door	Living room	Dining room	Kitchen	Laundry room	Bathroom	Bedroom	Closet	Home office	Garage	Exercise room	Outdoor areas
Equipment	High-spout faucet: provides extra clearance, making it easier to use				♦	♦	♦						
	Built-in shower seat: assists individuals who have difficulty standing for long periods						♦						
	Masonry walls: provide structural support, improve safety, prevent mold, and help retain heat						♦						
	Inverse or side-by-side refrigerator: provides easier access				♦								
	Lightweight furniture: facilitates movement		♦	♦				♦		♦			
	Appliance and equipment placement: should be functional for task performance				♦	♦							
Assistive technology	Simplified buttons: streamlined buttons improve device usability and efficiency. Integrate voice assistants for hands-free operation and programming of appliances				♦	♦							
	Intercom/communication system: reduces the need for long-distance movement	♦					♦						♦
	Automatic door closure (front door): prevents users from having to put down objects to close the door and helps in case of forgetfulness	♦									♦		
	Smoke sensor: prevents major fire-related accidents		♦	♦	♦	♦		♦	♦	♦	♦		
	Gas sensor: helps prevent accidents in case of gas leaks				♦	♦	♦				♦		
	Moisture sensor: alerts users to wet or humid areas						♦						

TABLE 17.1 *(Continued)*
Summary of Space Components for Safe Housing Environment

Categories	Guidelines	Front door	Living room	Dining room	Kitchen	Laundry room	Bathroom	Bedroom	Closet	Home office	Garage	Exercise room	Outdoor areas
Assistive technology	Motion-activated lighting: saves energy by automatically controlling lights or appliances. It provides convenience, enhances security, and supports accessibility while offering long-term cost savings and efficiency, especially at nighttime	♦	♦	♦			♦	♦	♦		♦	♦	
	Emergency alarm: assists in case of emergencies or hazards		♦	♦	♦	♦	♦	♦	♦	♦	♦	♦	♦
Constructive materials	Non-slip flooring: enhances grip during movement	♦			♦	♦	♦				♦	♦	♦
	Wood flooring: offers visual and environmental comfort; should have a matte finish		♦	♦				♦	♦	♦			
	Variety of furniture: allows different users with varying abilities, needs, and reach to use the same space		♦	♦									
	Water-resistant materials: prevent furniture degradation, reduce accident risks, and should be easy to maintain				♦	♦	♦				♦		♦
	Curtains: choose non-flammable materials. Avoid floor-length curtains and ensure they are easy to operate		♦	♦	♦			♦	♦	♦			
	Distinctive design: helps reinforce spatial recognition	♦											
	Small-tile flooring: increases the amount of grout, enhancing traction for the user					♦	♦						♦
	Visual communication: helps individuals to recognize their home and surroundings	♦											
	Outward-opening doors: prevents users from blocking the entrance in case of a fall in small spaces						♦						

TABLE 17.1 ***(Continued)***
Summary of Space Components for Safe Housing Environment

Categories	Guidelines	Front door	Living room	Dining room	Kitchen	Laundry room	Bathroom	Bedroom	Closet	Home office	Garage	Exercise room	Outdoor areas
Constructive materials	Heat-resistant surfaces: prevents breakage when placing hot objects				♦								
	Color contrast: helps identify environmental barriers	♦	♦	♦	♦	♦	♦	♦	♦	♦	♦	♦	
Furniture	Armchairs/chairs with armrests: provide secure support when sitting down or standing up		♦	♦	♦			♦		♦			
	Straight-legged tables and chairs: help prevent potential tripping hazards		♦	♦	♦					♦			
	Flexible layout: allows for adjustments based on user needs		♦	♦	♦					♦			
	Furniture positioned against walls: ensures unobstructed circulation		♦	♦				♦	♦	♦		♦	
	Firm mattress: assists with getting in and out of bed							♦					
	Drawer-style dishwasher: improves accessibility				♦								
	Use of drawers: enhances ease of use and accessibility, with handles designed as pulls to ensure a comfortable grip and smooth operation				♦	♦	♦	♦	♦	♦			
	Bench with armrests: provides a resting spot and assists with sitting down and standing up	♦											♦
	Table for support near the door: allows users to place objects while opening the door	♦											
	Mirror: enhances spatial perception and provides an expanded view of the environment, in addition to assisting with daily activities						♦	♦					
	Glass-door overhead cabinets: facilitate visibility of stored items				♦								

TABLE 17.1 *(Continued)*
Summary of Space Components for Safe Housing Environment

Categories	Guidelines	Front door	Living room	Dining room	Kitchen	Laundry room	Bathroom	Bedroom	Closet	Home office	Garage	Exercise room	Outdoor areas
Furniture	High cabinets: ideal to have a lift system to facilitate access to clothes. The cabinet doors, if present, can be made of glass to make it easier to see contents								♦				
Maintenence	Chemical storage: positioned within the user's reach envelope for safe access, stored away from gas sources or water contact, and kept out of children's reach					♦							
	Embedded wiring: loose cables create movement barriers. Avoid exposed wiring from floor lamps, table lamps, or small appliances		♦	♦	♦			♦	♦	♦			♦
	Efficient hinges and slides: facilitate smoother cabinet operation				♦	♦	♦	♦	♦	♦			
	Loose rugs: pose a physical barrier during movement, can accumulate dirt, and should be avoided		♦	♦	♦	♦	♦	♦	♦	♦			
	Low-maintenance finishes: make cleaning easier and faster, reducing the time and effort spent on upkeep	♦	♦	♦	♦	♦	♦	♦	♦	♦	♦	♦	♦

This information serves as a practical synthesis of the key elements explored throughout this book, offering a visually accessible and functionally organized tool for guiding design interventions. This summary reinforces the book's central message: designing safe, functional, and inclusive housing for older adults requires a systematic, evidence-based approach that considers not only physical safety, but also autonomy, dignity, and universal usability that meet the evolving needs of an aging population and benefit people across the life course.

18 Conclusions

Aging successfully is determined by a variety of factors, and the physical environment is an integral part of this process. The space in which one lives directly influences a person's ability to remain safe, autonomous, and engaged in activities of daily living. Designing safe and functional housing environments requires a multifaceted understanding of factors related both to the individual and the built environment. This involves recognizing the physical, cognitive, and sensory challenges older adults may encounter in using domestic spaces and, consequently, designing effective environments that not only enhance safety but also accommodate user limitations.

Furthermore, the emotional and psychological bond between individuals and their homes, commonly referred to as place attachment, is fundamental to aging in place. Homes must go beyond fulfilling only technical and functional requirements; they must also support the emotional, social, and psychological dimensions of older adults' lives. When thoughtfully designed, the physical environment contributes not only to safety and autonomy but also to one's sense of identity, belonging, and overall well-being. This book has been an effort to approach these complex issues through a structured and layered methodology.

In Section I, we introduced the theoretical and structural foundations that underpin design strategies for improving and adapting residential spaces. This theoretical basis is essential to provide a conceptual framework that informs and justifies design decisions. Without it, architectural and environmental interventions risk being arbitrary or misaligned with the real needs of the users.

In Section II, we transitioned from theory to application. Here, a practical and comprehensive analysis of all common residential environments was presented. For each space, specific strategies were proposed to guide the design of spatial components, categorized according to levels of safety priority. This prioritization system allows users—whether professionals, caregivers, or homeowners—to identify which elements are most critical, and thus prioritize certain interventions over others based on individual needs and available resources. Importantly, all the attributes and design features included in this section were drawn from scientifically grounded research. There may be other components worthy of consideration, but those selected for inclusion were those most consistently supported by empirical evidence. It is also essential to emphasize that when it comes to designing environments for older adults, projects must be genuinely user-centered. This means assessing the unique physical, cognitive, and emotional conditions of each individual. Understanding these personal circumstances is key to creating responsive environments that truly support independence, comfort, and quality of life. The contribution of this book, therefore, lies in presenting a flexible set of environmental features and design elements that can be adapted and customized depending on each user's particular demands.

In Section III, the book concludes with a general checklist designed to facilitate the application of the strategies presented throughout. This practical tool aims

DOI: 10.1201/9781003543701-21

to support professionals, caregivers, and older adults themselves in evaluating and improving their living environments with clarity and efficiency. Ultimately, the purpose of this book is to contribute to the improvement of people's lives by promoting safer, more inclusive, and more supportive living environments, especially for older adults. It advocates for housing solutions that go beyond minimum standards to foster dignity, independence, and well-being. In light of the global trend toward population aging, this is not only a professional challenge but also an ethical responsibility. It is our hope that the ideas presented here will serve as a valuable resource for anyone committed to designing homes that enable older adults to live not only safely but with purpose, autonomy, and quality of life.

Bibliography

CHAPTER 2

Lawton, M. P., & Brody, E. M. (1969). Assessment of older people: Self-maintaining and instrumental activities of daily living. *The Gerontologist*, *9*(3), 179–186. https://doi.org/10.1093/geront/9.3_Part_1.179

Lee, L. N., & Kim, M. J. (2020). A critical review of smart residential environments for older adults with a focus on pleasurable experience. *Frontiers in Psychology*, *10*, Article 3080. https://doi.org/10.3389/fpsyg.2019.03080

Nygren, C., Oswald, F., Iwarsson, S., Fänge, A., Sixsmith, J., Schilling, O., Sixsmith, A., Széman, Z., Tomsone, S., & Wahl, H.-W. (2007). Relationships between objective and perceived housing in very old age. *The Gerontologist*, *47*(1), 85–95. https://doi.org/10.1093/geront/47.1.85

Phillips, J., Walford, N., & Hockey, A. (2011). How do unfamiliar environments convey meaning to older people? Urban dimensions of placelessness and attachment. *International Journal of Ageing and Later Life*, *6*(2), 73–102. https://doi.org/10.3384/ijal.1652-8670.116273

Rogers, W. A., Meyer, B., Walker, N., & Fisk, A. D. (1998). Functional limitations to daily living tasks in the aged: A focus group analysis. *Human Factors*, *40*(1), 111–125. https://doi.org/10.1518/001872098779480613

Tomazzoni, A. M. R. (2011). A arte de morar só e ser feliz na velhice. *Kairós Gerontologia*, *13*(Especial 8), 109–123. https://doi.org/10.23925/2176-901X.2010v13iEspecial8p109-123

CHAPTER 3

Aihara, E. M. (2017). *Gestão de projetos habitacionais para idosos na cidade de São Paulo* (Trabalho de Conclusão de Curso, Escola Politécnica, Universidade de São Paulo). https://poli-integra.poli.usp.br/library/pdfs/0a00412d8182377fce4efa3d0a8f3d45.pdf

Bestetti, M. L. T. (2006). *Habitação para idosos: O trabalho do arquiteto, arquitetura e cidade* (Tese de doutorado, Universidade de São Paulo). https://www.teses.usp.br/teses/disponiveis/16/16131/tde-04032010-085452/

Bhidayasiri, R., Jitkritsadakul, O., Boonrod, N., Sringean, J., Calne, S. M., Hattori, N., & Hayashi, A. (2015). What is the evidence to support home environmental adaptation in Parkinson's disease? A call for multidisciplinary interventions. *Parkinsonism & Related Disorders*, *21*(10), 1127–1132. https://doi.org/10.1016/j.parkreldis.2015.08.025

Cruz, D. T. da, & Leite, I. C. G. (2018). Falls and associated factors among elderly persons residing in the community. *Revista Brasileira de Geriatria e Gerontologia*, *21*(5), 532–541. https://doi.org/10.1590/1981-22562018021.180034

Daré, A. C. (2010). *Design e ergonomia: Uma abordagem sobre a inter-relação entre o idoso e o ambiente doméstico*. Universidade Lusíada Editora.

Farber, N., & Shinkle, D. (2011). *Aging in place: A state survey of livability policies and practices*. AARP Public Policy Institute.

Hazin, M. M. V. (2012). *Os espaços residenciais na percepção dos idosos ativos* (Dissertação de mestrado, Universidade Federal de Pernambuco). https://doi.org/10.13140/RG.2.2.10577.17764

Lee, L. N., & Kim, M. J. (2020). A critical review of smart residential environments for older adults with a focus on pleasurable experience. *Frontiers in Psychology*, *10*, 1–15. https://doi.org/10.3389/fpsyg.2019.03080

Leiva-Caro, J. A., Salazar-González, B. C., Gallegos-Cabriales, E. C., Gómez-Meza, M. V., & Hunter, K. F. (2015). Connection between competence, usability, environment and risk of falls in elderly adults. *Revista Latino-Americana de Enfermagem*, *23*(6), 1139–1148. https://doi.org/10.1590/0104-1169.0331.2659

Lekić, O., Miletić, M., & Fikfak, A. (2018). Healthy places in the built environment. In A. Fikfak, S. Kosanović, M. Konjar, & E. Anguillari (Eds.), *Sustainability and resilience: Socio-spatial perspective* (pp. 217–232). TU Delft Open.

Lien, L. L., Steggell, C. D., & Iwarsson, S. (2015). Adaptive strategies and person-environment fit among functionally limited older adults aging in place: A mixed methods approach. *International Journal of Environmental Research and Public Health*, *12*(9), 11954–11974. https://doi.org/10.3390/ijerph120911954

Mace, R. (1998). *Universal design: Housing for the lifespan of all people*. U.S. Department of Housing and Urban Development. https://www.ncsu.edu/ncsu/design/cud/pubs_p/docs/housing.pdf

Manca, S., Cerina, V., & Fornara, F. (2019). Residential satisfaction, psychological well-being and perceived environmental qualities in high- vs. low-humanized residential facilities for the elderly. *Social Psychological Bulletin*, *14*(2), Article e33570. https://doi.org/10.32872/spb.v14i2.33570

Miguel, M. G. D., Moreira, M. A. S. P., Ferreira, O. G. L., Veloso, L. S. G., Silva, H. C., & Silva, A. O. (2018). Accidental falls involving elderly people: An integrative literature review/Acidentes por quedas em pessoas idosas: Um estudo de revisão. *Revista de Pesquisa: Cuidado é Fundamental Online*, *10*(4), 1188–1193. https://doi.org/10.9789/2175-5361.2018.v10i4.1188-1193

Phillips, J., Walford, N., & Hockey, A. (2011). How do unfamiliar environments convey meaning to older people? Urban dimensions of placelessness and attachment. *International Journal of Ageing and Later Life*, *6*(2), 73–102. https://doi.org/10.3384/ijal.1652-8670.116273

Porto, C. F., & Rezende, E. J. C. (2016). Terceira idade, design universal e aging in place. *Estudos em Design*, *24*, 152–168.

Ramadhani, W., & Rogers, W. A. (2022). Understanding home activity challenges of older adults aging with long-term mobility disabilities: Recommendations for home environment design. *Journal of Aging and Environment*, *37*, 341–363. https://doi.org/10.1080/26892618.2022.2092929

Romeiro, A., Almeida Prado, A. R., Besse, M., & Dutra, L. N. (2010). Moradia para o idoso: uma política ainda não garantida. *Kairós Gerontologia*, *13*(0), 5–17. https://doi.org/10.23925/2176-901X.2010v13i0p5-17

Van der Cammen, T. J. M., Albayrak, A., Voûte, E., & Molenbroek, J. F. M. (2017). New horizons in design for autonomous ageing. *Age and Ageing*, *46*(1), 11–17. https://doi.org/10.1093/ageing/afw181

CHAPTER 4

Fhon, J. R. S., Fabrício-Wehbe, S. C. C., Vendruscolo, T. R. P., Stackfleth, R., Marques, S., & Rodrigues, R. A. P. (2012). Quedas em idosos e sua relação com a capacidade funcional. *Revista Latino-Americana de Enfermagem*, *20*(5), 927–934. https://doi.org/10.1590/S0104-11692012000500015

Morais, H. C. C., Holanda, G. F., Oliveira, A. R. S., Costa, A. G. S., Ximenes, C. M. B., & Araujo, T. L. (2012). Identificação do diagnóstico de enfermagem "risco de quedas" em idosos com acidente vascular cerebral. *Revista Gaúcha de Enfermagem*, *33*(2), 117–124. https://doi.org/10.1590/S1983-14472012000200001

Morsch, P. (2017). *Desenvolvimento de um instrumento para avaliação da percepção do risco de quedas em idosos* (Tese de doutorado, Pontifícia Universidade Católica do Rio Grande do Sul). https://tede2.pucrs.br/tede2/handle/tede/7533

Index

Note: Page numbers in *italics* indicate a figure.

R

S

U

www.ingramcontent.com/pod-product-compliance
Ingram Content Group UK Ltd.
Pitfield, Milton Keynes, MK11 3LW, UK
UKHW022211190926
475702UK00003B/309

* 9 7 8 1 0 3 2 8 9 6 1 8 2 *